THE QUAKER HERITAGE IN MEDICINE

By

Robert A. Clark, M.D.

and

J. Russell Elkinton, M.D.

THE BOXWOOD PRESS

Second Printing, 1986
With minor additions.

Distributed by

The Boxwood Press
183 Ocean View Blvd.
Pacific Grove, CA 93950

ISBN: 0-910286-68-X

Printed in U.S.A.

PREFACE

ON April 9 and 10, 1976, the Friends Medical Society, a small informal group of doctors and health workers who are members of the Religious Society of Friends, held a Bicentennial symposium in Philadelphia. The subject of the symposium was the Quaker heritage in medicine and its application to the problems of today. What was there in the religious backgrounds, beliefs, and experiences of Quaker workers in the fields of physical and mental health that, in the past, contributed to their professional effectiveness? And what value might this Quaker heritage have in meeting the health problems of today?

To help to characterize this Quaker heritage the undersigned presented to the first session of the symposium two historical papers: one on Quakers and psychiatry and one on Quakers in medicine. These papers, amplified and rewritten, are the material of this book. They are published here in the hope that a wider audience might share some of the information, interest, and inspiration that came to the authors as they explored, however briefly, the lives and accomplishments of certain of our Quaker forerunners in the arts and sciences of healing.

Of necessity, these brief surveys provide more historical breadth than depth. We can name and discuss only a limited number of the many Friends engaged in medical activities over the three centuries from George Fox and his contemporaries to our own contemporaries of the present day. We hope that our choices are not invidious and that our readers will forgive us for seemingly unwarranted omissions. But within these limitations we have tried to convey the sweep of Friendly concern for physical, mental, and spiritual health that is our Quaker heritage in medicine, a heritage with which we face the future.

Robert A. Clark, M.D.
J. Russell Elkinton, M.D.

August 1978

Contents

Part I

QUAKERS AND PSYCHIATRY

By

Robert A. Clark, M.D.

Staff Psychiatrist
Friends Hospital

Clinical Professor of Psychiatry (retired)
Hahnemann Medical College

Friends Hospital, Philadelphia, PA 19124

Introduction

THIS PART deals with the Quaker concern for the care of the mentally ill. It is a concern not well known among most Quakers, though very familiar to those who have studied the history of psychiatry. It should be more widely known, and deserves to be studied as an example of the usefulness of individual and corporate effort in alleviating one of the commonest and least understood forms of human suffering.

This concern began very soon after the Society of Friends was founded. In 1649, according to George Fox's *Journal,* two healing meetings for worship were held for the benefit of a mentally sick woman. At the second meeting "about the first hour the Life rose on Friends . . . and she was well" (Pickvance, 1957). In 1669 Fox advised Friends to provide "a house for them that be distempered" (Braithwaite, 1921). In 1671 London Quakers were seeking a suitable place in or about their city for Friends who might be "distracted or troubled in mind, that so they may not be put amongst the world's people or run about the streets." Dr. ***John Goodson,*** a surgeon of London, provided a large house for their reception and care. Though John Goodson emigrated to America soon after, we do not hear that he continued his interest in the insane.

The Eighteenth Century

Quaker Concern for the Insane in Colonial America

AMONG the supporters of Dr. Thomas Bond and Benjamin Franklin in founding the Pennsylvania Hospital in Philadelphia in 1751, however, were many Quakers. Provision of medical care for the insane was one of the primary reasons for its founding. In the library at Friends Hospital is a book entitled *The History of the Pennsylvania Hospital, 1751-1895* (Morton and Woodbury, 1895). It is of interest to those concerned with the history of psychiatry in Philadelphia, because much of it has to do with the care of the insane before Friends Hospital opened in 1817. For Quakers it is of special interest, since many of those involved in the early management of Pennsylvania Hospital were of that persuasion.

One such Quaker was Israel Pemberton, Jr. The grandson of a companion of William Penn and the son of one of the wealthiest merchants of his time, he was active in establishing the Hospital and was a member of the first Board of Managers in 1751. He had several other concerns. An earnest and true friend of the Indians, familiarly called "King Wampum," he accompanied others in 1756 to a conference at Easton with the Delawares and other Indians. He was a founder of the Friendly Association for Regaining and Preserving Peace with the Indians by Pacific Measures. He was twice arrested for the criticism of the authorities: once by Governor Thomas Penn, and once in 1777 because of his disapproval of the Revolutionary War. He was dispatched to Staunton, Virginia, for the latter offense without a trial, together with his brothers, James and John, and other dissident Friends, and remained there eight months. He died in Philadelphia in 1779. Three other Quaker exiles who were on the Board were Edward Pennington, Thomas Fisher, and Thomas Wharton.

It is not surprising that Israel Pemberton was among the signers of the original petition to the House of Representatives of Pennsylvania for the establishment of the Hospital. Benjamin Franklin wrote the petition and was also a member of the 1751 Board of Managers. Other Quaker names appear among the signers and the Board: Evans, Reynell, Shoemaker, Rhoads, Smith, and Allen. John Smith, of the first board, married a daughter of James Logan, Penn's secretary. He helped in raising money in the early years by sending letters soliciting funds to foreign correspondents he knew through his shipping and importing business. Israel and

James Pemberton also gave financial help by borrowing the first 1000 pounds received from the Pennsylvania legislature, engaging to repay it whenever building was decided upon.

Several Friends were among the early physicians at the Hospital. ***Cadwalader Evans*** was appointed in 1759. ***Caspar Wistar,*** professor of anatomy at the University of Pennsylvania Medical School, was a Friend. ***Thomas Chalkley James*** was a descendant of a celebrated Quaker preacher, Thomas Chalkley of Frankford. The only direct connection with Friends Hospital was through Dr. ***Samuel Emlen.*** He graduated from the University of Pennsylvania in medicine in 1812, and served as physician to the Friends Asylum

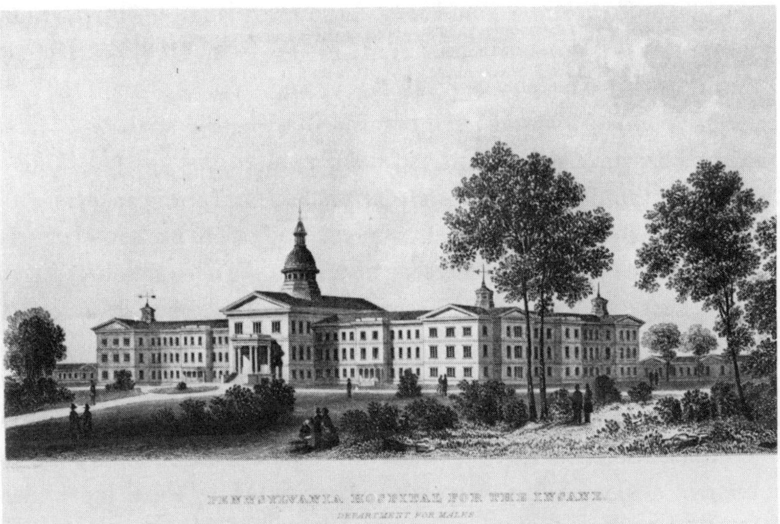

Pennsylvania Hospital for the Insane, about 1840.

for the Insane before his election to Pennsylvania Hospital's medical staff in 1823. He was active in organizing the Pennsylvania Society for Discouraging the Use of Ardent Spirits.

We cannot claim ***Benjamin Rush*** as a Friend. However, his ancestors were, coming to Pennsylvania in 1683. Many of his principles accorded with those of Quakers. He advocated temperance, condemned the use of tobacco, and opposed capital punishment. Though an ardent supporter of the Revolution, he was fruitful with ideas for universal peace. He was president of the American Society for the Abolition of Slavery. Concern for the care of the mentally ill was his chief professional interest.

The most active Friend on the Hospital's Board in these early years was ***Samuel Coates.*** An orphan, he was raised by his uncle, John Reynell, a member of the Board in 1752. In 1785 Coates himself was elected a Manager. Right away he was appointed to a committee to report on "a plan of economy and on the cause of the great expense of the house." When yellow fever struck in 1793, he was the only manager found at his post in Philadelphia throughout the epidemic. When another epidemic arose in 1798, he sent his family out of the city and, as he wrote, "took up my abode in Pennsylvania Hospital." He continued with this anecdote: "One night I dreamed the Prisoners [at the penitentiary] would make a violent attempt to rush out." He left the hospital after breakfast and waited on Robert Wharton, the mayor, and offered to send Francis Higgins, the Hospital steward, to his aid. Wharton refused this help. Less than five minutes after the refusal, several prisoners tried to escape.

Samuel Coates kept a diary for many years, recording observations relative to the hospital, including the behavior of the insane patients. Shortly before his death in 1830, he presented his diary to Benjamin Coates, his son, who was trained in medicine under Dr. Philip Physick. Benjamin Coates gave the address at the laying of the cornerstone of the Department for the Insane at 49th and Market streets in 1836.

Before the opening of this institution in 1840, the mentally ill were housed in the Hospital, first at the temporary quarters on Market Street and then for many years on Pine Street. One of the purposes of founding the Hospital was to take care of "lunatics or persons distempered in mind," so that "they may be restored to reason and become useful members of the community"—a hopeful outlook. Of the two patients admitted on the first day the doors were open on February 11, 1752, one was insane.

In the beginning their treatment was not entirely in accordance with the principles of humanity later practiced at Friends Hospital and the Hospital's own Department for the Insane. Acute cases, so-called "Phrenzy," were "douched . . . alternately with warm and cold water, their scalps were shaved and blistered; they were bled to the point of syncope; purged, and, in the intervals, chained by the waist or the ankle, to the cell wall." In 1752 orders were placed with

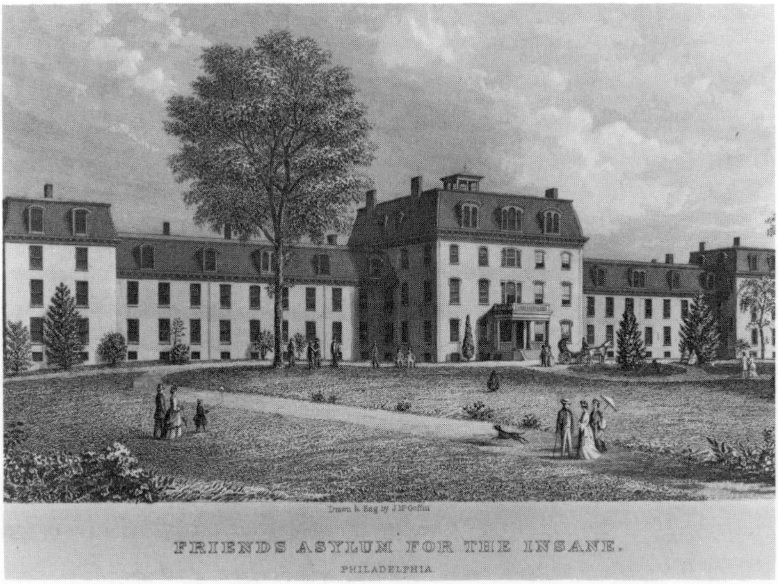

Friends Asylum for the Insane, Philadelphia, after 1875.

the blacksmith for handcuffs, leg locks, rings, staples, and "swifells" for leg chains. Soon efforts were made by the Managers to better conditions. In 1756 and 1762 the basement cells were improved to prevent dampness and discourage rats. Samuel Rhoads and others were appointed to this task. In 1784 an attempt was made, for the first time, to heat the rooms in winter with charcoal braziers in the corridors, the only effect being near suffocation of keepers and patients alike. Not until 1833 were the rooms adequately warmed. In 1760 concern was expressed over idle and curious people who gathered around the windows to look at the patients, or to tease and annoy them. Samuel Rhoads and his committee were asked to build a fence before the windows and otherwise control the public.

In his diary Samuel Coates recorded a number of interesting and pitiful cases of mental illness among the patients. One Quaker woman, Hannah Lewis, showed evident signs of her illness by preaching in Friends Meeting, on the Court House steps, and in other public places. Calling herself a daughter of King George the Second, she went to London as a stowaway to visit the royal family. She was permitted to walk in the queen's garden. Her funds exhausted, she returned to Philadelphia and was finally admitted to Pennsylvania Hospital. She remained there for 17 years, until her death at 89.

Pennsylvania Hospital for a number of years had treated its mental patients with considerable humanity under the direction of Dr. Benjamin Rush, the first American physician who can with justice be called a psychiatrist, and a student of the works of the great French reformer, Dr. Philippe Pinel.

In 1818 ***Samuel Mason,*** a Friend and steward of the Hospital, wrote in a letter concerning the care of the insane there: "I have not the most distant doubt but kindness in every instance has a more happy effect than contrary treatment, and when coercion is resorted to, still to endeavor to impress on their minds that it is for their good and not to gratify any resentment that punishment is inflicted. Their memory is generally acute, and kindness remembered: also any unkind image is not soon forgotten" (Mason, 1951).

Early Quaker Care of the Insane in England

ONE MUST return to England for the further history of Quaker concern with the mentally ill. In 1790 a Quaker named Hannah Mills was confined in York Asylum. She died within a few weeks.

Her relations and friends were not permitted to visit her on the grounds that she was not in a suitable state to be seen by strangers. A number of members of York Meeting soon after were moved to consider the propriety of founding an establishment for the care of their mentally ill. Among the founders was ***William Tuke,*** a tea merchant, descendant of an earlier William Tuke who was a follower of George Fox. The senior Tuke died in 1669 after twice suffering imprisonment for his beliefs. In March 1792 the junior

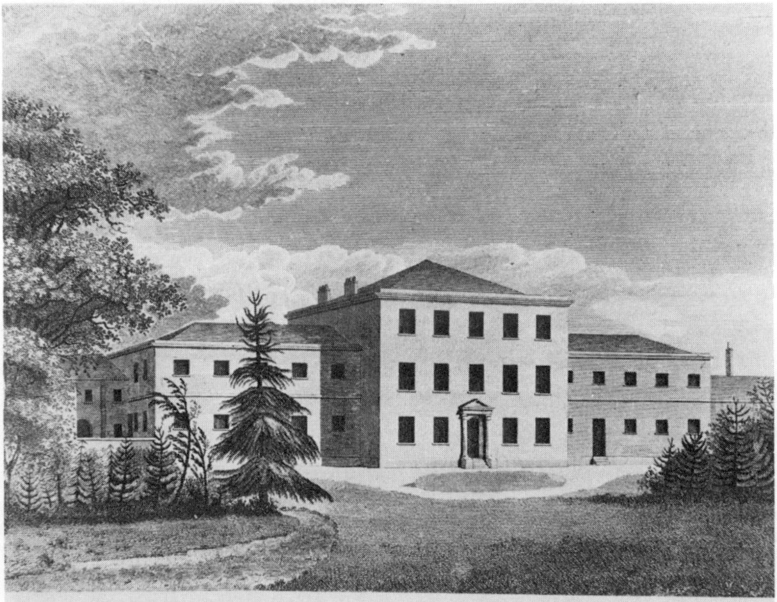

PERSPECTIVE VIEW of the NORTH FRONT of the RETREAT near YORK.

Tuke laid a proposal before the Quarterly Meeting of Yorkshire for a "retired habitation . . . for the members of our Society and others in profession with us, who may be in a state of lunacy, or so deranged in mind as to require such a provision" (Hunt, 1932). A subscription was at once begun. On May 11, 1796, the Retreat at York opened its doors. They have not been closed since.

From the beginning, drugs and medicines, then so often used in excess, were found to be of little benefit. More effective were warm baths, liberal diet, suitable amusements, and reading—except, of course, "works of imagination," or, as we now call them, novels. Neither chains nor corporal punishment was permitted, and mechanical restraint was seldom used. Those more violent were separated from the more tranquil. Fresh air and gardening were prescribed. Many patients attended Friends meeting in the city. The superintendent read the Bible to most of the patients on Sunday afternoons; the reading was followed by a period of silence, even among those "much disposed to action." Such was the "moral treatment of the insane" as begun in this quiet place.

The York Asylum heard more of the Retreat in 1813. ***Samuel Tuke,*** William's grandson, published that year his *Description of the Retreat.* Alarmed, Dr. Charles Best, the superintendent of the Asylum, accused Tuke of defamation. In October Samuel Tuke and twelve other leading citizens went to a meeting of the governors, paid their dues, and forced the setting up of a committee of inquiry. In August 1814 every officer, keeper, and nurse was removed, and Dr. Best resigned. The managers of the Retreat took over the running of the Asylum until a new staff was found.

In May 1814 a similar committee of Londoners visited Bethlem Royal Hospital. What they found led to the appointment of a parliamentary committee which inquired into Bethlem, the York Asylum, workhouses, and private "madhouses" throughout England. Their report appeared in 1815, followed in the next two years by reports on the conditions of the "lunatic poor" in Scotland and Ireland. Not until 1828 were acts of Parliament passed amending the laws of 1774 regarding the erection and regulation of county asylums. Meanwhile, conditions at Bethlem had much improved (Macalpine and Hunter, 1963).

Few Friends realize that the Retreat at York was not the first English institution founded by a Friend for the treatment of the mentally ill. When William Tuke was looking for a matron to care for the female patients at the Retreat, he found a capable person in Katherine Allen, an employee at Cleve Hill near Bristol, a private hospital maintained by Dr. ***Edward Long Fox.*** A graduate from medical school in Edinburgh, Dr. Fox lived from 1761 to 1835 and was described as the sire of a long line of "mad doctors" (Hunter and Macalpine, 1963). He directed Cleve Hill from 1794 to 1806. He was on the staff of Bristol Royal Infirmary from 1784 to 1816. In 1804 he opened a new asylum, Brislington House, in Bristol. One learns something about this place from an account written by its best-known patient, John Thomas Perceval, concerning his own treatment there in 1831 and 1832 (Bateson, 1961). Perceval was a son of Spencer Perceval, prime minister, who was assassinated in the House of Commons in 1812. While at Oxford University in 1830, John Thomas was severely conflicted on the subject of religion. Hearing of some religious enthusiasts in Scotland, reputed to speak in tongues, he went to Edinburgh to see them. Evidently the turmoil between his conscience and his own sense of sin was too much for him, for in January 1831 he was taken to Brislington House. He remained there until May 1832. His observations concerning Dr. Fox, then 70, reflected his estimate of his own social standing, if nothing else.

> Dr. Fox had been a member of the Society of Friends. The spirit of the burlesque doctrines of that sect crept into his system. When I complained of the degrading footing of familiarity on which I had been placed with the domestics, he replied "Had not Jesus made us all equal?" The servant whom I used to call Jesus, ran with me, jumped, joked, walked arm in arm with me. This conduct may be partly accounted for by having been placed under a quondam Quaker, to whom perfect equality of rich and poor was a matter of faith.

Fox was among the first licensed house proprietors to practice humane methods based on the abolition of restraint on so large a scale. In Parry-Jones's opinion, "his achievements seriously rival those of Samuel Tuke" (Parry-Jones, 1972). In 1828 he was called to give evidence before the Select Committee of the House of Lords. In 1829 he gave up the management of Brislington House to two of his sons, Drs. F. K. and C. J. Fox. The average number of patients there was about 90.

Edward Wakefield, a Quaker who combined his business travels as a land agent with philanthropic tours of asylums in England, gave evidence in 1815 before the Select Committee. He testified that Fox's establishment was "delightfully and cheerfully situated." Though a Quaker, Fox was the first private proprietor to introduce regular religious observances according to the Church of England, paying a salary to a local clergyman who officiated at the asylum chapel. His primary intention was to reproduce patterns of normal social activity.

According to Wakefield, little or no coercion was used, and the benefit of occupation, amusement, and exercise was stressed. The example set by Dr. Fox, another observer stated in 1816, illustrated the fact that "brutal treatment of lunatics was unnecessary." Conditions at Brislington House contrasted with those Wakefield found in the ward for incurable lunatics at Guys Hospital in London, where he saw two patients lying naked in straw and where conditions remained unsatisfactory until the ward was closed in 1861. Brislington House, Parry-Jones wrote, "adopted methods of treatment, as advanced as those at the York Retreat, although they never enjoyed the publicity gained by the latter."

In the eighteenth century many American Quakers traveled to England. One was John Woolman of Mount Holly, New Jersey, who came to York in 1772 and died there of smallpox. He was buried in an unmarked grave in York. Henry Tuke, William's son, was so influenced by John Woolman that he was led "to feel a deeper interest in the wrongs of the slave and in other subjects with which the tender, self-sacrificing mind of the messenger had been occupied." We are not told of his influence on William himself. In 1784 a New York Quaker, Lindley Murray, settled in York because his doctor had told him that a cool climate was good for the chronic illness from which he suffered. He lived there until his death in 1826, having published a grammar, speller, and a book of French selections which secured his renown among the teachers of the English-speaking world. When he died, he left 25 English pounds "to the Lunatic Asylum" (Frank, 1826).

See page 78 for an account of a Quaker Hospital in Ireland.

Expansion of Care for the Mentally Ill

WHEN *Thomas Scattergood,* a Quaker minister of Philadelphia, visited York in 1799, he dined with Lindley Murray and was taken to visit the Retreat. Returning to York seven months later, he first found lodging with Lindley Murray, and on successive days dined with Henry and William Tuke. He then "felt a concern to go to the Retreat, a place where about 30 of our Society are taken in, being disordered in mind. We got most of them together, and after we had sat a little in quiet, and I had vented a few tears, I was engaged in supplication." This experience must have touched him deeply (*Journal of Thomas Scattergood,* 1874).

Scattergood was unquestionably moved by an incident that occurred in 1808 while he was going from Downingtown to Lancaster in Pennsylvania. He and several companions stopped at a Friend's house for the night. "It was truly a house of mourning," his memoirs relate. "The wife of their host had long been in a desponding condition of mind. Thomas Scattergood was introduced into deep sympathy with the poor distressed woman, and the next morning, he gave vent to his religious exercise on her account." The memoir continues, "At the time of the ensuing Yearly Meeting a woman Friend greeted Thomas Scattergood with affectionate animation, and, she exclaimed, 'Why, doesn't thee know me? I am the Friend that through thy instrumentality was raised right up out of the earth.' She continued in a sound mind, and was afterwards appointed to the station of an Elder, and was esteemed as a valuable Friend" (*Memoirs of Thomas Scattergood,* 1844).

Three years later, in 1811, proposals were made to the Philadelphia Yearly Meeting "to make provision for such of our members as may be deprived of the use of their reason." In 1812 a plan was agreed upon, subscription papers drawn up, and the distribution committed to seven Friends. The first name on the list was that of Thomas Scattergood. A general meeting of the subscribers was held on April 14, 1813. Land was bought later in the same year, in Frankford, now part of the city of Philadelphia. On May 15, 1817, the first building was opened for patients; it is still in use. Unhappily Thomas Scattergood had died in 1814, but his son Joseph was a member of the original Board of Managers. There have been several members of the Scattergood family on the Board of Friends Hospital since.

A book that was used to encourage Friends in Philadelphia to contribute to the new institution was Samuel Tuke's *Description of the Retreat at York,* published in 1813. His book circulated throughout Great Britain, the continent of Europe, and America, and did much to acquaint physicians and others with the principles to guide men in the treatment and care of the insane.

One of those who read Samuel Tuke's book was ***Thomas Eddy,*** a member of the Board of Governors of New York Hospital in New York City (Russell, 1945). He was a Quaker merchant, a tireless worker for human welfare. With others he had endeavored to prevent the increase of taverns in the city. He had been an inspector for seven years of the state prison he had helped to found. During this time he had introduced industries into the prison. He conducted them so efficiently that their profits in the last year of his service equaled the cost of the prison's operation. He was also active in establishing the Bible Society, the Free School Society, and Manumission Society (for buying the freedom of slaves), the Savings Bank, the Society for the Reformation of Juvenile Delinquents, and the Humane Society. As governor of the Hospital since 1793, he was largely instrumental in obtaining funds for establishing a separate department in the hospital in 1808 for the care of the insane. He was a member of the first Asylum Committee.

When a man who showed such unremitting concern for so many new advances in social welfare read a book like Samuel Tuke's, it did not take him long to act. On April 4, 1815, Eddy presented at a special meeting of the New York Hospital Board a carefully prepared plan based on his "perusing the works of Benjamin Rush, but more particularly the account of the Retreat near York," and proposed that ground be purchased for a separate and rural institution for the "moral management" of the insane. The governors appointed Thomas Eddy, John Murray (Lindley's nephew), and others to purchase the land. On August 1, 1815, 38 acres were bought at Bloomingdale, near the present location of Columbia University.

Thomas Eddy had written to Lindley Murray that same year about his plans. Murray had replied that he was "putting thy pamphlet and letter into the hands of my benevolent and zealous friend, Samuel Tuke." A letter dated July 17, 1815, was received from Tuke, enclosing a floor plan to a new asylum at Wakefield, England. With this help, plans progressed rapidly. The cornerstone of Bloomingdale Hospital was laid on May 7, 1818. The new institution was opened in 1821, with Thomas Eddy as chairman of the Asylum Committee. This hospital was the immediate predecessor of the Westchester Division of the New York Hospital in White Plains, New York, one of the leading private nonprofit mental hospitals in the United States.

An early resident physician who served at Friends Hospital from 1832 to 1833 was ***Thomas Kirkbride.*** He was a young Philadelphia Quaker and a graduate of the University of Pennsylvania Medical School. When Pennsylvania Hospital wished to open its own separate institution for the insane in West Philadelphia, Thomas Kirkbride was invited to be its superintendent. The first patients arrived on January 9, 1841. "Moral suasion" was Kirkbride's chief principle. Mechanical restraint was rarely used. One day when 104 patients were in the hospital, only one patient was in restraint, and for ten days thereafter, none. In 1842 Kirkbride wrote,

> The value of employment in the treatment of insanity is now universally conceded. The object is to restore mental health and tranquilize the restlessness and mitigate the sorrows of disease. Drawing and painting were taught by an artist from the city. Several patients gave instructions to others on the same ward in different branches of learning, these were lectures on astronomy, electricity, physiology, optical illusions, and the wonders of nature and of Egypt. (Bond, 1947)

Thomas Kirkbride often worked closely with others who shared his principles. The most notable reformer of his day in the care of the mentally ill was Miss Dorothea Lynde Dix, a retired Massachusetts school teacher and a Unitarian. She first became aware of the abuses of the treatment of the insane when, on going to the state prison in Boston to teach a Sunday School class, she found a number of mentally ill confined there. For years afterward she traveled about this country and abroad, inducing legislatures to found new mental hospitals and urging the improvement of those already existing. In 1844 she came to Pennsylvania and met Kirkbride. The next year he wrote to her, promising to help further the establishment of a state hospital at Harrisburg, the capital of Pennsylvania. They often corresponded in the years following.

On October 15, 1844, Kirkbride invited twelve other hospital superintendents to his home for dinner. They came from Massachusetts, from Virginia, and from intervening states. The next day, at a meeting in Jones Hotel in Philadelphia, the Association of Medical Superintendents of American Institutions for the Insane was founded. This was the parent organization of the American Psychiatric Association. Thomas Kirkbride was its first secretary and later its president.

In 1854 the first edition of his book, *On Hospitals*, was published, embodying his ideas on hospital architecture. In later years this book was used in planning new mental hospitals by 31 states from Connecticut to California. The Kirkbride plan can still be seen exemplified in mental hospital buildings throughout the country.

One of Dr. Kirkbride's guests at dinner in 1844 was Dr. ***Pliny Earle*** (Sanborn, 1898). He had been born in 1809 in Leicester, Massachusetts, the scion of an old Quaker family. After graduating from medical school in Philadelphia, he was resident physician at Friends Hospital from 1840 to 1844. He then took charge of Bloomingdale Hospital which Thomas Eddy had done so much to found. There he began the statistical study of mental illness. He was a great traveler. Before going to Friends he had been in Europe, visiting the Tukes at York and meeting Elizabeth Fry in England. In

Paris he visited the Bicêtre, the Salpêtrière, and other hospitals. He even inspected a mental institution in Constantinople. There he found all the patients but one in chains, and that one locked in a room for 15 years. All these patients, nevertheless, appeared to be in good physical health and were often visited by their physician. Ten years later, in 1849, after leaving Bloomingdale, he toured Germany and Austria, visiting their mental institutions. Earle had published in 1841 an account of the varied conditions he found in hospitals he had visited, from the most enlightened to the most medieval (Earle, 1841).

A new state hospital was opened in 1858 at Northampton, Massachusetts. In 1864 Pliny Earle became its superintendent. The remainder of his professional life was spent at Northampton. There he continued his statistical studies, which led to his celebrated work on the curability of the insane. With the utmost sanity, he punctured the inflated claims of some of his colleagues to have cured in one year more patients than had been admitted to their hospitals that same year! They had simply counted many patients twice or more—particularly alcoholics—because they had been admitted and discharged more than once in the same year. This bit of Quaker common sense brought to the statistics of mental illness high standards which have prevailed ever since.

Earle's successor as resident physician at Friends Hospital was Dr. ***Joshua Worthington*** (Dain, 1964). In 1850 he became the first physician to be the Hospital's superintendent. He kept the position until 1877. Worthington held steadfast for moral treatment at a time when pessimism increasingly prevailed—a pessimism encouraged by the rising belief in organic causes of mental illness and by the overcrowding in state hospitals due to heavy European immigration. He insisted on psychological predisposing causes: lack of religious education and of training in morality and self-control, lack of useful vocational training, and violent fluctuations in the business world. In the 1840s Dr. John Conolly had instituted a policy of nonrestraint into his hospital at Hanwell, England. Though Pliny Earle had been somewhat skeptical of the value of this policy, Joshua Worthington introduced it into Friends Hospital in the 1850s.

In 1852, spurred on by Dorothea L. Dix, President Fillmore and Congress authorized the establishment of a federal hospital for the insane in the District of Columbia. The president appointed as its first superintendent. Dr. ***Charles H. Nichols,*** who had been a resident physician since 1849 at Bloomingdale Hospital. Charles Nichols's birth place was Vassalboro, Maine. He attended the Friends School in Providence, Rhode Island, and graduated in medicine at the University of Pennsylvania in 1843.

From 1847 to 1849 he was trained in psychiatry at the Utica State Hospital in New York under Dr. Amariah Brigham, another of Dr. Kirkbride's dinner guests in 1844. The institution in Washington (now St. Elizabeth's Hospital), built under Nichols's direction, was modified from Kirkbride's architecture. Nichols's modifications were adopted by many American state hospitals and in institutions in Newfoundland and Australia. A lodge for the Negro insane was probably the second such provision ever made for that race. Appointed superintendent of Bloomingdale Hospital in 1877, Nichols traveled in Europe to study new psychiatric methods preparatory to moving that institution to its new setting in White Plains. He was president of the Association of American Superintendents of Institutions for the Insane. A leading forensic psychiatrist, he testified in defense of Guiteau, the assassin of President Garfield. His biographer states, "No doubt his interest in [the mentally ill] was due to his upbringing among the Quakers" (*The Dictionary of American Biography,* 1927).

In 1853 a Quaker merchant of Baltimore applied to the Maryland legislature for a charter for a new mental hospital in that state. This man was ***Moses Sheppard*** (Forbush, 1968; 1971). He had been born in Montgomery County, Pennsylvania, about 1772. Because his father was a Tory, the family went to Nova Scotia when Moses was still an infant. Soon after they returned and settled near Baltimore. His parents having died while he was still a boy, Moses went to work to support himself. Within a few years he

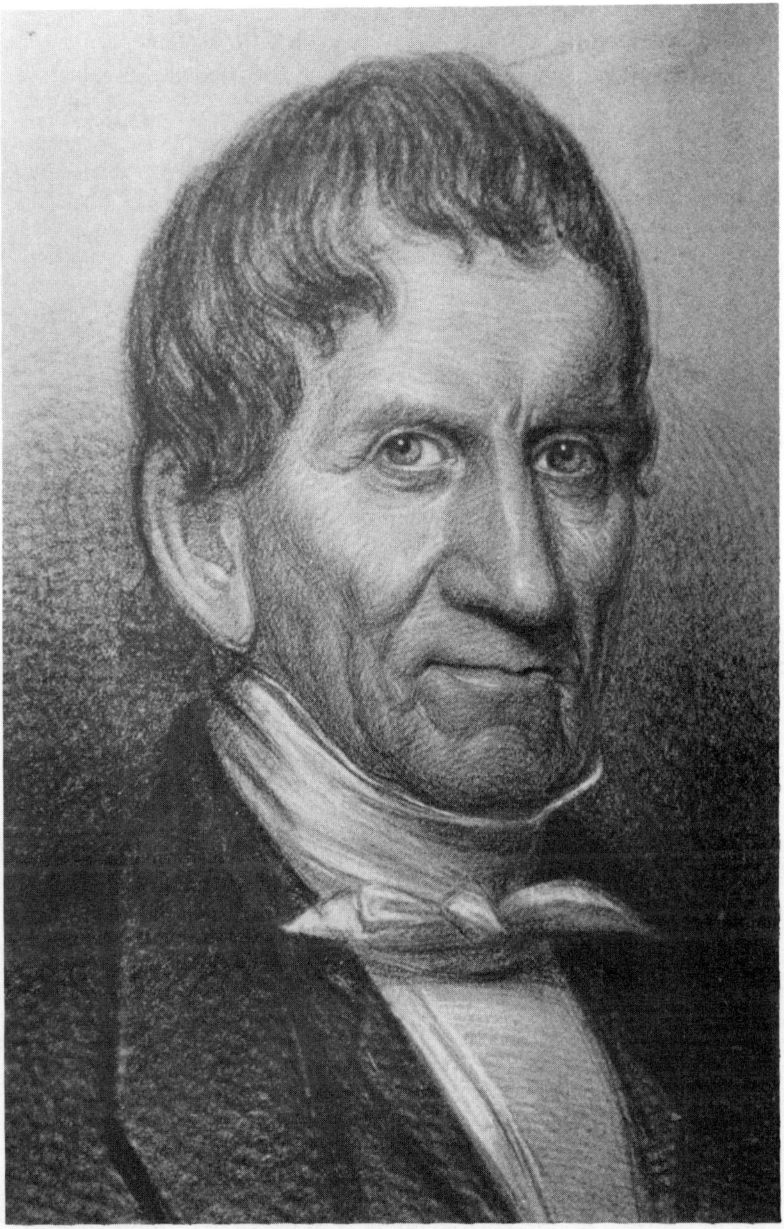

Moses Sheppard (1772-1857)

became a very successful textile manufacturer. In the 1830s he was much interested in colonization of Negroes in Liberia.

On March 19, 1853, he wrote to his good friend, Dr. Nathan Shoemaker:

> There is a strong movement here to complete a juvenile house of reformation and erect two hospitals for the insane and I expect what I may leave will take that direction and not to individuals. It had been stated in England, that more of the Society of Friends became insane, in proportion, than of any other Society or class; I don't know if it is so or not, but there are several here; and more of us half-crazy.

It is not known whence came Sheppard's concern with the care of the insane. A letter written in 1843 told how his friend Henry Payson became a physical and mental invalid, "the remnant of body and mind," and object of pity, "whose mind is gone; he looks at me with a vacant, idiotic stare painful to the beholder." Sympathy for this friend may have led to his later generosity.

Moses Sheppard announced his intention that his hospital would be

> experimental, a small establishment for the poor only. The institution was intended in the first instance for the members of the Society of Friends of which I belong. Quakers are never found in the Almshouses, and they have been compelled for the want of an Insane Asylum of their own to send their patients to such Institutions abroad. They have but one Institution for the Insane, a small one, near Philadelphia. My object is to establish a similar one here.

Before his death in 1857, he appointed several Friends to the Board of Managers.

He left nearly his whole fortune, almost $600,000, for the care of the institution. The year following, an estate of 375 acres was bought at Towson, just outside Baltimore. Construction was delayed because the will did not permit the principal to be touched. In fact, it was not until after another large bequest had been received from Enoch Pratt, founder of the public library of Baltimore, and a Unitarian, that the hospital was finally completed and opened in

1891. Since then it has maintained a high reputation under the name Sheppard and Enoch Pratt Hospital. The majority of its board are still Quakers. That Quaker influence is still strong can be judged by the fact that when a new recreation building was opened in 1958, it had attached to it a small wing containing a Quaker meeting house.

Samuel Tuke, the author of *Description of the Retreat,* had two sons who were concerned Friends. The younger, ***Daniel Hack Tuke,*** was the first psychiatrist in his family. Born in York in 1827, he studied medicine in London and Heidelberg. Following his graduation, he was physician at the Retreat for several years. He traveled extensively on the Continent, visiting mental institutions and meeting the leading psychiatrists of his day. He was editor of the *Journal of Mental Science,* Britain's chief psychiatric journal, from 1880 until 1895. He wrote numerous books on various subjects such as hypnotism, the history of psychiatry in Britain, and the influence of the mind on the body. He visited the United States and Canada. When Dorothea Dix was in England, she spent some time as his guest. Daniel Hack Tuke was unquestionably one of the greatest psychiatrists of his time. With his death in 1895, the dynasty of Tukes ended after almost a century of work in British psychiatry and of influence extending far beyond their own land (Zilboorg, 1941).

Quaker Psychiatry in the Twentieth Century

IN the twentieth century Quaker psychiatric hospitals have continued their service. Many Quaker psychiatrists, other mental health workers, and laymen have been members of their staffs and boards of managers. On the occasion of its 100th anniversary in 1913 the name "Friends Asylum" was changed to "Friends Hospital," and an historical volume was issued. Friends Hospital has just erected a new building named after William Tuke. The 75th anniversary of Sheppard and Enoch Pratt Hospital was celebrated in 1967. The addresses given on the occasion were published (Gibson, 1967). Bliss Forbush, a Friend, chairman of the Board for a number of years, wrote a biography of Moses Sheppard and a history of the Hospital, which are among sources for this article. Harry Stack Sullivan and Lawrence S. Kubie, who were research psychiatrists there, wrote many books and papers, especially on schizophrenia.

At the time of World War II, many Friends and others similarly minded in the United States worked in mental hospitals and institutions for the retarded as conscientious objectors on alternative service (Clark and Burgess, 1948). By 1942, these institutions were in desperate need of personnel. Selective Service, the American Friends Service Committee, the National Committee for Mental Hygiene, and the superintendents of several institutions collaborated in arranging for conscientious objectors to volunteer to work as attendants. Many grasped the chance—approximately 4000 throughout the war. Most of the units in state hospitals were administered by religious bodies, 20 by the Mennonite Church, 8 by the Brethren, 6 by the Religious Society of Friends, 3 by other denominations. Other conscientious objectors worked in schools for the retarded and in veterans' psychiatric facilities.

The conscientious objectors soon recognized how inadequate many of the institutional services were, not only because of war shortages, but to some extent by financial, administrative, and professional deficiencies existing before the war. They talked and wrote to each other, trading information and ideas. Soon they organized the Mental Hygiene Program of Civilian Public Service, got out a monthly magazine called *The Psychiatric Aide,* and began to agitate for improvement. They wrote articles, or supplied information to reporters, for newspapers and magazines, and solicited the support of prominent psychiatrists and laymen. They helped to draft a model law for the commitment and care of the mentally ill.

Perhaps the most effective action was taken in Ohio. A reporter for the *Cleveland Press* wrote a series of articles regarding conditions reported to him by conscientious objectors at a nearby state hospital. D. R. Sharpe, a Baptist minister, led a grand jury investigation and helped revitalize the Ohio Mental Hygiene Society. The conscientious objectors were discharged from the hospital, then reinstated. Eventually the state hospital system was reorganized under new leadership, with larger legislative appropriations. This instance, though more dramatic than most, is in the tradition of Samuel Tuke's actions at the York Asylum in 1813.

Many concientious objectors continued their interest in mental health after peace came. Some studied to become psychiatrists, psychologists, or social workers, among them a number of Friends. Some became active in founding the National Mental Health Foundation, later merged with the National Association for Mental Health. The work of all these men had some influence in the later founding of psychiatric clinics and the development of comprehensive mental health centers in the 1950s and 1960s. They helped to staff these new providers of psychiatric care, both as professional workers and as administrators.

It is worth noting that many conscientious objectors worked at Friends Hospital, Sheppard and Enoch Pratt Hospital, and other psychiatric institutions during the Vietnam war.

Individual Friends who have contributed much to psychiatry in recent years may be mentioned. Dr. Erich Lindemann, author of a landmark paper on grief (Lindemann, 1944), taught at Harvard Medical School, practiced at Massachusetts General Hospital, and helped organize a pioneer mental health center in Massachusetts. Dr. William P. Camp was superintendent of Norristown State Hospital and Commissioner of Mental Health of Pennsylvania, later director of Friends Hospital. Dr. Douglas Hitchins was the subject of an article in the *Friends Journal* (Cattell, 1976). In addition to his being clerk of New York Monthly Meeting, he has been staff chairman of a Quaker committee on heroin addiction and chairman of the Friends Conference on Religion and Psychology. The late Dr. Robert E. Jones was clinical director of the Instituite of the Pennsylvania Hospital and a student of the life of Benjamin Rush.

The Conference on Religion and Psychology was initiated more than 25 years ago by Klined Kotchnig, a psychologist, Jungian analyst, and a Friend. She was editor of its official journal, *Inward Light*. The conference meets annually at Haverford College, near Philadelphia. A number of Quaker psychiatrists and psychologists have been active participants. Dr. Leon Saul, psychoanalyst and psychiatric consultant at Swarthmore College, for example, one year spoke on the topic of aggression.

For a number of years Philadelphia Yearly Meeting has sponsored a family relations counseling service, staffed by Quaker social workers and psychologists. Two psychiatrists have been consultants, Dr. Ross Roby and Dr. Howard Wood. Roby was a conscientious objector during World War II, with alternative service at Philadelphia State Hospital. Later he was the child psychiatrist at Northeast Community Mental Health Center, which has its headquarters on the grounds of Friends Hospital. Wood has taught psychiatry for some time at the University of Pennsylvania School of Medicine.

In 1976 the Superintendent of the Retreat at York was an Irish Friend, Dr. John O'Neil Gillespie. He and his wife were guests that year at the dedication of the William Tuke building at Friends Hospital.

Characteristic of Quaker concern with mental and emotional problems is the fact that psychiatrists and laymen have worked together. In the early days there were lay-superintendents of hospitals. Now there are Quakers who are board members, administrators, volunteers, fund raisers, and mental health workers of several kinds. Laymen and professional workers share the idea that there is a "divine spark" in everyone, no matter how clouded by illness or defect; there are no elite patients. As Edward Long Fox said, "Jesus made us all equal." The best available care should be the right of all, not a privilege for the few. Over the centuries those most likely to be neglected by our government and society have especially concerned the Friends—the mentally ill, as well as prisoners, minorities, dissidents, the aged, and the poor. Friends have always had an interest in education, as well, both for their own members and for others. Their institutions have become centers for teaching and training. They have traveled throughout the world in order to find out how the mentally ill are cared for. It is hoped that these traditions will continue. The understanding and the treatment of mental and emotional problems will remain one of the principal interests for many members of the Religious Society of Friends.

SELECTED REFERENCES

Bate. , Gregory, ed. *Perceval's Narrative: A Patient's Account of His Psychosis, 1830-1832.* Stanford, Calif.: Stanford University Press, 1961.

Bond, Earl D. *Dr. Kirkbride and His Mental Hospital.* Philadelphia: Lippincott, 1947.

Braithwaite, William C. *The Second Period of Quakerism.* London: MacMillan, 1921.

Cattell, Elizabeth. "Douglas Hitchings." *Friends Journal* 22(1976):173.

Clark, Robert A., and Alex M. Burgess, Jr. "The Work of Conscientious Objectors in State Mental Hospitals during the Second World War." *Psychiatric Quarterly Supplement* 22(1948):128.

Dain, Norman. *Concepts of Insanity in the United States, 1789-1865.* New Brunswick, New Jersey: Rutgers University Press, 1964.

The Dictionary of American Biography. "Charles H. Nichols." New York: Scribners, 1927.

Earle, Pliny. *A Visit to Thirteen Asylums for the Insane in Europe.* Philadelphia: J. Dobson, 1841.

Forbush, Bliss. *Moses Sheppard: Quaker Philanthropist of Baltimore.* Philadelphia: Lippincott, 1968.

———. *The Sheppard and Enoch Pratt Hospital, 1853-1970.* Philadelphia: Lippincott, 1971.

Frank, Elizabeth. *Memoirs of the Life and Writings of Lindley Murray.* York (England), 1826.

Friends Asylum for the Insane, 1813-1913. Philadelphia: Winston.

Gibson, Robert W., ed. *Crosscurrents in Psychiatry and Psychoanalysis.* Philadelphia: Lippincott, 1967.

Hunt, Harold C. *A Retired Habitation: A History of the Retreat.* London: H. K. Lewis, 1932.

Hunter, Richard, and Ida Macalpine. *300 Years of Psychiatry, 1535-1860.* London: Oxford University Press, 1963.

Journal of Thomas Scattergood, Philadelphia, 1874.

Lindemann, Erich. "The Symptomatology and Management of Acute Grief." *American Journal of Psychiatry* 101(1944):141.

Macalpine, Ida, and Richard Hunter. *George III and the Mad Business.* New York: Pantheon, 1969.

Mason, Samuel. "Pennsylvania Hospital in 1818." *American Journal of Psychiatry* 108(1951):384.

Memoirs of Thomas Scattergood, vol. 8. Philadelphia: Friends Library, 1844.

Morton, Thomas, and Frank Woodbury. *The History of Pennsylvania Hospital, 1751-1895.* Philadelphia: Times Printing House, 1895.

Parry-Jones, William L. *The Trade in Lunacy.* Toronto: University of Toronto Press, 1972.

Pickvance, Joseph. "George Fox, Healing and Spiritual Regeneration." *Friends Quarterly* 11(1957):8.

Russell, William L. *The New York Hospital: A History of the Psychiatric Service.* New York: Columbia University Press, 1945.

Sanborn, F. B. *Memoirs of Pliny Earle, M.D.* Boston: Damrell and Upham, 1898.

Zilboorg, Gregory. *A History of Medical Psychology.* New York: W. W. Norton, 1941.

Part II

QUAKERS IN MEDICINE

By

J. Russell Elkinton, M.D., M.A.C.P., F.R.C.P.

Emeritus Professor of Medicine
University of Pennsylvania

Editor Emeritus, *Annals of Internal Medicine*
American College of Physicians

Colwall, Herefordshire, England

Introduction

FOR three hundred years members of the Society of Friends have been seekers of the "abundant life." Believing that God, the Supreme Power in the Universe, is good and that some portion of his power lies as an "inner light" or "spark" within each human being, Quakers have ever attempted to cultivate this spark to the end that the lives of all men might be creative, mutually beneficial, and satisfying. It is not surprising, therefore, that many members of the Society, concerned over the illnesses—physical, mental, and spiritual—that beset their fellow men, felt called to practice the healing arts. From the early days of faith healers and apothecaries, of doctors of physick and chirurgeons, to the complex personnel of the present day, physicians and surgeons, psychiatrists and psychologists, nurses and pharmacists, physiotherapists and social workers, Quakers have served with devotion and distinction in these professional capacities. Three centuries of such service have bequeathed to us a Quaker heritage in medicine.

Quakers in medicine have no monopoly in compassion or the desire to serve; over the same centuries physicians of many faiths and religious beliefs have shared in upholding the Hippocratic code and in maintaining the profession's tradition "to cure sometimes, to relieve often, to comfort always." What then may distinguish the Quaker doctor as such and what may be unique about the Quaker heritage in medicine? It was to try to answer these questions that this study was undertaken.

THE STUDY BEGINS with a survey of the lives of certain Quaker doctors in various stages of the history of the Society of Friends. It deals primarily with individual people rather than with organizations, programs, or committees (to which the Society is much addicted). Physicians and surgeons mainly are considered because of the limitations of time and space; the role of other health workers is not meant to be minimized. Psychiatrists and other workers with the mentally ill (a field in which Quakers have been distinguished pioneers) have been largely left to the pen of Dr. Robert

Clark in the accompanying paper. Finally, this survey is directed in the main to cover Quakers in medicine in, and from, Great Britain; those in America and elsewhere in the world, although they share the common heritage, will have to await a further study. Within these limits, we will examine briefly, century by century, the lives of Quaker doctors for their medical and scientific activities, their broader social concerns, and, where known, their religious interests. In so doing, we will look for the effect of their Quakerism on their professional activities and, in turn, for the effect of these Quaker doctors on the medical profession. Herein surely must lie the character of the Quaker heritage in medicine.

ONE MORE WORD about the reasons for attempting to delineate this particular Quaker heritage at this particular time. The world of today is a very different world from that of George Fox three hundred years ago. The scientific and technological revolution has given man enormous powers to alter, for better or for worse, the quality of his own life and that of the planet. Growing out of this revolution are enormous problems: the threats of increased violence and of nuclear holocaust, of overpopulation and famine, of maldistribution of resources, of ecological damage to the environment, of social and political disruption, of moral decay. But science has also given man increasing ability to understand his world and these problems contained in it, and to understand himself. However, science alone is not enough; men and women everywhere are searching for the power of the spirit to help them meet the multiple challenges to the quality of their lives. Within this context both the individual patient who is ill and the individual physician and healer face critical problems. The patient finds adequate health care ever more difficult to obtain and he has a sense of diminishing personal contact with, and understanding by, his doctor. The physician has much greater knowledge of the workings of the human body, of the causes of disease, and of effective ways to treat them; but likewise his difficulties are many. He finds it harder to keep up with the advances of medical science, he knows that many of these more powerful treatments may produce undesirable or even dangerous side effects or may lead to agonizing moral and ethical dilemmas. Increasingly he is aware that most patients need treatment not only of their bodies but of their minds and their spiritual lives as well. Does the Quaker heritage in medicine speak to these conditions of this present age?

Second Half of the 17th Century

The Beginning of Quakerism

THE RISE OF QUAKERISM from the preachings of George Fox began in mid-century during the Cromwellian inter-regnum and, after the restoration in 1660 of Charles II and the Stuart monarchy, flourished despite severe persecution by the strongly Anglican Parliament. But it was not a period when men of learning who were dissenters found it easy to pursue their professions. Of the Quaker doctors and healers in this initial period of the Society of Friends we know relatively little. Our inquiries begin, quite literally, with George Fox.

George Fox (1624-1691). Although the founder of the Society was not trained in medicine, he was said to be an herbalist of considerable skill. In addition, we now know that he was an extraordinarily effective faith healer, with a record of some 150 "miraculous" cures. These cures were recorded in George Fox's *Book of Miracles*, but shortly after his death this record was suppressed by the Society for fear of embarrassment. However, an index of the work survived and most of the cases have been reconstructed from the clues of this index by that astute sleuth in the field of Quaker history, Henry J. Cadbury. These reconstructed cases he published in 1948 along with a fascinating commentary on Fox's relations with the medical profession of the time. George Fox's "patients" came mainly from the poor and humble folk among whom he moved, and the diseases cured included such nonspecific conditions as "lameness," "scrofula," and "sores." Henry Cadbury judged that only 18 of the 150 conditions cured were primarily mental in character; the rest seemed to be physical ailments that improved remarkably after George Fox's ministrations of healing.

These ministrations of healing, however, were not confined to the spiritual; apparently George Fox was adept at physical manipulation as well. In his *Journal* he describes, during his religious journey in the American colonies in 1672, how he saved the life of his companion, John Jay of Barbados, who, when thrown from his horse, appeared to be quite lifeless with a broken ("loose") neck. George braced himself against a log, seized John's head, and pulled and twisted it until the neck became firm and John began to breathe again. "So we bound up his neck warm with a napkin" and the following day John Jay rode horseback 16 miles to the next meeting "and many hundreds of miles afterwards through the woods and the bogs." This was a therapeutic result that surely would satisfy any orthopedic surgeon or osteopath today.

Nevertheless, George Fox was not opposed to regular practitioners of medicine and was on good terms with Quakers who were doctors. One of these, especially close to Fox, was ***Thomas Lower***, who, as husband of a daughter of Margaret Fell, became Fox's stepson-in-law. Dr. Lower shared with George Fox his long imprisonment in Worcester and there Fox dictated to him part of his autobiography. Another Quaker physician was "Dr." ***Edward Bourne*** of Worcester, probably an apothecary, with whom Fox traveled in 1656 and who remained his friend for years. But Fox did not hesitate to try to keep his medical friends up to scratch with his query (that time-honored Quaker method of upholding standards):

> All you that be physicians and doctors, have you the wisdom by which all things was made? Have you the knowledge of the virtue of all things in creation?

The profession would be hard pressed to live up to this standard even in the 20th century.

Some of the Quaker doctors of this period were men trained on the Continent, especially in Holland and Germany, who joined

Friends after emigrating to England. These included ***Albertus Otto Faber, Francis Mercurius van Helmont,*** and ***Henry Lampé.*** Dr. van Helmont is best known for his position as family physician to a famous Quaker patient, Lady Conway of Ragley Hall. Dr. Lampé was a Huguenot who, after he joined Quakers, practiced first in York and then in Ulverston. In addition, there must have been many other doctors of physick, chirurgeons, and apothecaries who on becoming Quakers continued in their professions. Henry Cadbury has found evidence that several groups of such doctors met together to examine the meaning of their new faith for their occupation. One such group met in the home of James Wasse, chirurgeon, in London in 1683, and another "Chirurgeons Meeting" was held in 1679 in Barbados (where a large proportion of the local doctors were Quakers). Perhaps these groups were the first forerunners of our present-day Friends Medical Society.

Charles Lloyd (1637-1698) and ***Thomas Lloyd*** (1640-1694). These two brothers from Dolobran in Montgomeryshire, Wales, read medicine at Oxford shortly before their conversion to Quakerism. They were landed gentry, and when their father died prematurely, Charles left the university to take over the family estate. He married Elizabeth Lort from distant Pembrokeshire and soon after the birth of their first son joined the Quakers in 1662. Immediately he and a number of other Friends in the area were thrown into prison in Welshpool where his wife joined him the next year. This imprisonment—later mitigated by parole from the common gaol to a house in the town—lasted 10 years and during this time three more children were born to them. Charles Lloyd apparently never practiced medicine, but he was a leading member of the Society of Friends and became the progenitor of the long line of Quaker Lloyds renowned as ironmasters, businessmen, and bankers in the Midlands and especially in the rising industrial city of Birmingham.

Meanwhile Thomas Lloyd, on hearing of the imprisonment of his brother, left Oxford to assist his sister-in-law in looking after the Dolobran estate. In 1663 he, too, joined Quakers. As he was not imprisoned, he not only worked to help his coreligionists and spread Quakerism but also developed an active practice of medicine. In 1683 Thomas Lloyd, with his wife and children, emigrated to Pennsylvania. In the new settlement of Philadelphia he rapidly became a leading Quaker figure and a close friend of William Penn. He served as deputy governor during part of the long period that Penn was absent from the colony. At the same time Thomas Lloyd continued to practice medicine in a pioneer community that periodically was ravaged by such diseases as yellow fever and malaria. His wife and some of his children died (including his son), but today there are in Philadelphia many descendants of his daughter Nancy. We know little detail of Thomas Lloyd's activities as a physician and surgeon, but he surely deserves a place in the history of Quaker medicine on both sides of the Atlantic.

Thomas Lloyd was not the only doctor in William Penn's new colony: other medical Quakers from Wales and England came with Penn. These included ***Thomas Wynne*** of Flintshire, ***Edward Jones*** of Bala, ***Griffith Owen*** of Lancashire, and ***Robert Dimsdale.*** These Quaker chirurgeons, along with ***John Goodson,*** who had come over before Penn, and physicians ***Hugh Chamberlain, Charles Marshall,*** and ***William Russell*** began the practice of medicine in Pennsylvania.

Comment

The first generation of Quakers of George Fox's time were mainly yeomen-farmers and people in the humbler walks of life. As such, their medical problems must have been to a large extent dealt with by home remedies and beyond that by the services of herbalists, apothecaries, midwives, and perhaps faith healers. The healing services of George Fox fitted well into these patterns. Qualified doctors of physick and chirurgeons, such as they were, received their professional training either in England before they left the established church (as did the Lloyd brothers), in Scotland, or on the Continent, whence they came and joined the Society of Friends (as did Drs. Faber and van Helmont). Whatever the extent of their professional training, these early Quaker healers had a deep religious faith in the power of the indwelling God that directed their ministrations to the spiritual, as well as to the physical, needs of those who sought their aid. They treated the whole man.

The Eighteenth Century

The Age of Enlightenment

THIS WAS THE AGE in England when men of broad interests and independent minds began to seek scientific knowledge and apply it to industry; it was the time of the active growth of the Royal Society in London and of the similar but smaller Lunar Society in Birmingham. Many Quakers of inquiring mind shared in these activities and not a few of them were medical men. For the Society of Friends it was a period of lessened persecution and of greater economic stability deriving from integrity and ingenuity applied to commerce and industry. Quakers as dissenters were still denied entrance to Oxford and Cambridge. Friends who aspired to practice medicine still apprenticed themselves to apothecaries and physicians, but an increasing number extended their medical education by attending the medical schools in Edinburgh and Leyden. Such Quaker doctors played their full share in the development of 18th century science as well as medicine.

John Fothergill (1712-1780). John Fothergill was clearly the outstanding Quaker doctor of his century. Born into a Quaker family in Yorkshire (his father John and his brother Samuel were Quaker ministers well known in both England and America), he was apprenticed to the Quaker apothecary ***Benjamin Bartlett*** of Bradford and subsequently completed his medical training in Edinburgh and Leyden. He then settled in London where he became one of its most eminent physicians of the latter half of the 18th century. His medical skill was great and his practice was enormous, ranging from the poorest in the city to the aristocracy.

But John Fothergill was much more than a practicing physician; the scope of the medical, scientific, social, religious, and political activities of this extraordinary man was astounding. He studied epidemic (diphtheritic and streptococcal) sore throat, scarlet fever, tuberculosis, and smallpox. He recognized that poverty and squalor contributed to the diseases that he saw and so campaigned for more sanitary water supplies, prison reform, and better social conditions

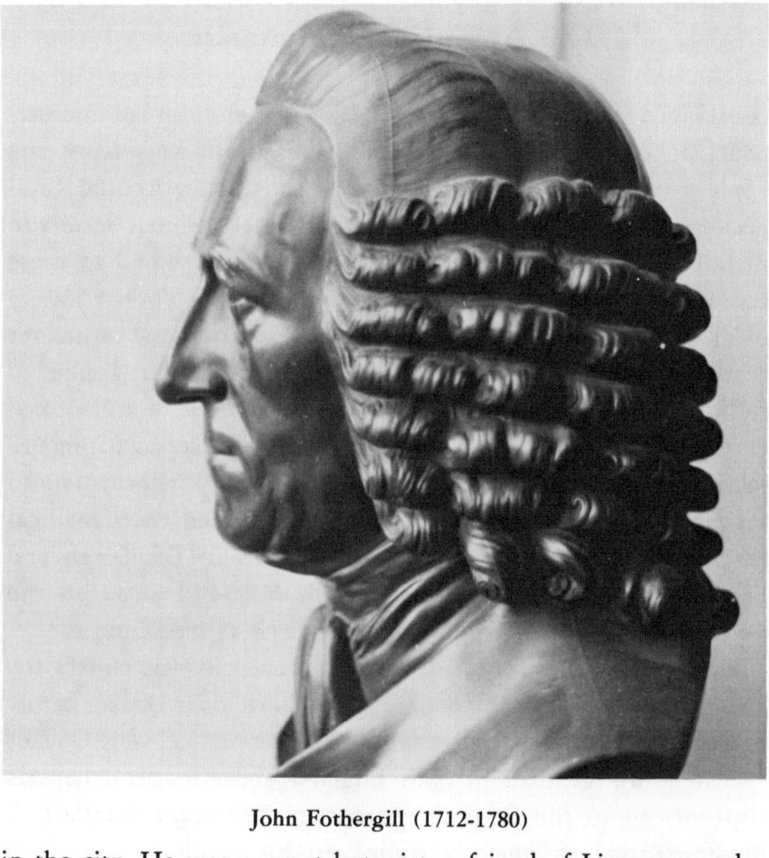

John Fothergill (1712-1780)

in the city. He was a great botanist, a friend of Linnaeus, and a Fellow of the Royal Society; and through collectors in many parts of the world he created the finest botanical garden in the England of his day. He was a pillar of the London Yearly Meeting of the Society of Friends, of which he was three times clerk, and he corresponded extensively with members of the Society in America. With his friend, Benjamin Franklin, he tried very hard, but unsuccessfully, to divert the British government of Lord North from military confrontation with the American colonies.

John Fothergill was an educator. He founded Ackworth School, one of the earliest Quaker boarding schools. He was active in the Royal College of Physicians of London and helped to start the forerunner of the Medical Society of London. He encouraged Benjamin Franklin and Dr. ***Thomas Bond***, Quaker physician, to found the Pennsylvania Hospital in Philadelphia, contributing some of the first books and funds to this earliest hospital in the American colonies. Perhaps his greatest medical influence was a personal one on young physicians, many from America, who were entertained in his home and counseled as to their medical studies. Among these especially to be noted were Dr. ***Benjamin Waterhouse*** of Rhode Island, a young American cousin of his, who was to become the first professor of physic at Harvard; and Drs. ***John Morgan***, ***William Shippen, Jr.***, and ***Benjamin Rush***, all of whom were responsible later for starting the first American medical school at the University of Pennsylvania. Dr. Fothergill continued his active interest in the new Pennsylvania Hospital and so influenced, at least indirectly, other Quaker doctors on the staff. These included not only Dr. Thomas Bond but his brother Dr. ***Phineas Bond***, as well as Drs. ***Thomas Cadwalader***, ***Lloyd Zachary***, and ***John Redman***, who became the "grand old man of the medical profession in Philadelphia" in his time and the first president of the College of Physicians of Philadelphia.

John Fothergill was a man of pleasing personality, liberal in his ideas, fond of young people, compassionate to patients, and generous to all. As a man and as a physician, he left an indelible mark on medicine.

John Coakley Lettsom (1744-1815). Here was another able and versatile doctor, the special protegé of Dr. Fothergill who succeeded him as the leading Quaker physician in London. Lettsom was one of a seventh pair of twins born to Quaker parents on Tortola in the

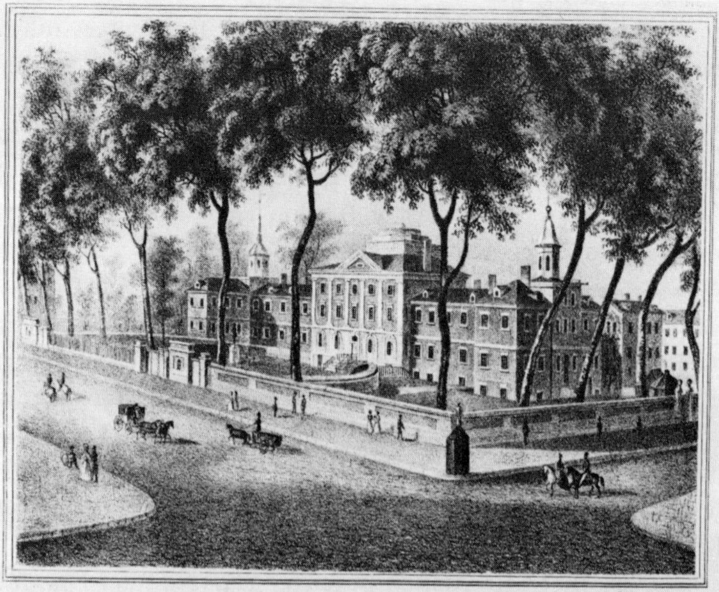

PENNSYLVANIA HOSPITAL

PHILADELPHIA.

Entered according to act of Congress in the year 1838 by J T Bowen in the Clerk's Office of the District Court for the Eastern District of Penn^a

British West Indies. Because the previous six pairs had all died of "tropical fever," he was sent as a small boy to Lancashire to be raised under the care of the Fothergill family. He was apprenticed to the Quaker apothecary ***Abraham Sutcliffe*** of Settle, studied medicine at Edinburgh, and then practiced in London. He had a keen mind for medical studies and promoted the use of inoculation and, after Jenner, vaccination for the prevention of smallpox. He was the principal founder of the prestigious Medical Society of London that exists to this day. Like his mentor John Fothergill, he was sensitive to the social and medical needs of the time, and with Fothergill he established a series of free public dispensaries for the poor of the city. The two physicians also set up a line of rescue stations along the Thames riverside to apply the new technique of resuscitation to drowning persons; this system eventually became the Royal Humane Society. In his later years Lettsom decided that the poor and sick in the city would benefit from sea air and sea bathing, and to this end he established a center for sea bathing in Margate. In addition to all these medical activities, he too was an ardent botanist and collector with a fine botanical garden around his home in Camberwell. And he was an enthusiastic mineralogist whose collection eventually formed the core of the mineral collection at Harvard. He was a Fellow of the Royal Society. John Coakley Lettsom deserves to be remembered for more than a rhyming pun on his name.[1]

Thomas (Baron) Dimsdale (1712-1800). Thomas Dimsdale was another Quaker doctor who was a friend of John Fothergill. When the latter was asked by the Empress Catherine of Russia to come to that country to inoculate her son against smallpox, Dr. Fothergill sent Thomas Dimsdale in his stead. Prior to Jennerian vaccination with cowpox, inoculation with live smallpox virus carried a substantial risk of mortality; in this instance, the inoculator was at risk as well as the inoculatee. Nevertheless, Dr. Dimsdale carried out the procedure successfully on both the empress and her son and was rewarded with a large sum of money and the title of baron. He returned to London where he confined his practice to immunizing against smallpox. He is said to have rather fallen away from the Society of Friends as he enjoyed the worldly advantages of his fame, fortune, and title.

There were, of course, numerous other Quaker doctors of the 18th century; many of them had interests outside their medical work but only some of them can be noted here. ***Gilbert Thompson*** (1726-1803) was a younger kinsman and protegé of John Fothergill. He was a quiet, unassuming man, something of a classical scholar, who practiced in London, and was the author of one of the first memoirs of John Fothergill after the latter's death. Two other

1. Contemporary caricature in verse of Dr. Lettsom's vigorous therapeutics:

When any sick to me apply,
I physics, bleeds and sweats 'em
If after that they choose to die,
Why verily!
I Lettsom

Quaker medical men were also botanists and as such were closely associated with Lettsom: ***William Curtis*** (1746-1799),[2] apothecary, and ***William Woodville*** (1752-1805), physician, who wrote a five-volume work on medical botany as well as supervised the Smallpox Hospital of St. Pancras. ***Thomas Knowles*** (1734-1786), like John Fothergill, was born in Yorkshire and became a leading Quaker physician in London; in 1783 he was appointed to the first Quaker committee concerned with the abolition of slavery in British territories. ***Robert Willan*** (1757-1812), also born in a Quaker family in Yorkshire, came to practice in London at the suggestion of John Fothergill and became the founder of dermatology in England. He was a fine classical scholar, a student of the Gospels, and an advocate of public-health measures for the poor. ***John Rutty*** (1698-1775), from a Quaker family in Wiltshire, studied medicine under Boerhaave in Leyden, was another friend of John Fothergill, and for many years was a prominent practitioner in Dublin. His scientific interests centered around hydrology and the relation of weather to disease; his religious convictions as a Quaker were strong: he was an elder, kept a spiritual diary, and wrote a history of Quakers in Ireland. ***George Vaux*** was a Quaker chirurgeon in London and was one of the group of doctors who helped John Lettsom in establishing the new free public General Dispensary. ***George Birbeck*** (1776-1841) was yet another Quaker physician from the Yorkshire Dales; he was born in Settle, received his M.D. in Edinburgh in 1799, and subsequently practiced in London. Here he founded the London Mechanics Institution that grew into the present-day Birbeck College of the University of London. He, too, served in the General Dispensary. One should not forget among the Quakers in the London medical world the apothecaries ***Silvanus Bevan*** (1691-1761) and his younger brother ***Timothy Bevan.*** These two brothers, sprung from a Quaker family in South Wales, were admitted to the Society of Apothecaries, became Fellows of the Royal Society, and from their premises in Lombard Street

2. This William Curtis, "The Botanist," was a member of the fourth of six generations of Quaker doctors in the Curtis family of Hampshire; in the fifth generation was Dr. William Curtis (1803-1881), "The Naturalist," of Alton.

developed a high reputation for providing pure drugs at a fair price—so much so that Dr. John Fothergill engaged them to supply the first shipment of drugs to the new Pennsylvania Hospital in Philadelphia. Subsequently, the Bevan family trained a young apothecary, ***William Allen*** (1770-1843), who eventually took over the firm. Allen combined great talents as a scientist (he was chemist at Guy's Hospital and was elected Fellow of the Royal Society) and as a Quaker philanthropist. From his home and shop in Plough Court he launched the first Peace Society, traveled widely in support of the movements to improve prison conditions and to abolish slavery, and in later years founded the Lindfield colony to provide education and industry for agricultural workers.

Three more Quaker doctors of this century are of interest because of their connections with America. ***William Hillary*** (1697-1763) practiced in Ripon, Yorkshire, but went out to the Barbados where in 1751 he treated Lawrence Washington, the older brother of George Washington, and was the first to describe the disease of tropical sprue. ***William Small*** (1734-1775) began his professional life as professor of mathematics at the William and Mary College in the colony of Virginia where Thomas Jefferson was his student and friend. Subsequently he came to Birmingham, England, to practice medicine, where he became a member of the Lunar Society. Here he used his engineering skills to patent a one-wheel clock and to assist James Watt and Mathew Boulton in the development of the steam engine. A third versatile young Quaker doctor was ***William Thornton*** (1761-1828) who, like John Coakley Lettsom, was born of English Quaker parents on Tortola in the British West Indies. Lettsom became his patron and sent Thornton to study medicine in Edinburgh, Aberdeen, and St. Bartholomew's in London. He returned to North America and practiced medicine in Philadelphia and on Tortola. However, he is most famous for his avocation of architecture; in 1789 he won the competition for the design of the new capitol of the United States to be built in the proposed city of Washington. Thus he became a close companion of President Washington and was one of the first commissioners of the new capital city.

No account of the Quaker contribution to 18th century medicine can omit mention of the enlightened treatment of the insane. The story of the establishment in 1796 of the Retreat at York by the Quaker businessman ***William Tuke*** (1732-1822) is told in Part I by Dr. Clark.

Comment

Quaker doctors of the 18th century were true members of the "age of enlightenment." Many of them were "polymaths" whose inquiring minds and scientific interests ranged over the entire field of human knowledge. They shared in the growing activities of the Royal Society and the Lunar Society, activities that underlay the start of the Industrial Revolution. But these men did more. As members of the Society of Friends, their religious concern for all people led them beyond conventional medical practice to instigate practical measures to combat the social wrongs that undermined the health of the people. To this end they promoted better sanitation, established public dispensaries, gave freely of their skills to indigent patients, organized to meet the emergencies of accidents and drownings, advocated prison reform. And not least, they promoted education: general education—as in the founding of Ackworth School—and medical education—as in the establishment of societies to foster medical knowledge and in the counseling of young physicians, many of whom came from the American colonies. Finally, these Quaker doctors were active members of the Society of Friends and often served as clerks, elders, and ministers. Polymaths indeed!

Early and Mid-Nineteenth Century

The Industrial Revolution and Quaker Quietism

THE FIRST part of this century saw the era of quietism in the Society of Friends. Quakers tended to be turned in on themselves and to concentrate on their business activities. Businesses expanded, the Industrial Revolution accelerated with the building of the canal systems followed by the railways; Quakers were closely involved in these developments. At the same time Parliament became open to Friends and subsequently, in 1871, the universities of the Establishment—Oxford and Cambridge. In mid-century, modern medical science really began as the discipline of pathology (or morbid anatomy) flourished and the discoveries and practices of bacteriology were applied to human diseases. To these developments Quaker doctors and scientists were major contributors. A few of the outstanding Quaker medical men may be noted.

Thomas Young (1773-1829). Born into a Quaker family in Somerset, Thomas Young was a child prodigy who became an "English Leonardo." Not only did he study medicine, he was as well a classical scholar, a philosopher, a linguist, a philologist, and a student of physics. He studied medicine at St. Bartholomew's Hospital and then practiced in London where he taught at the Middlesex Hospital and St. George's Hospital. He was a pioneer in the field of ophthalmology, being the first to describe the physiology of accommodation and color vision; for these contributions he was elected to the Royal Society. Among his nonmedical contributions were formulations of theories of mechanics and energy that were forerunners of concepts in the field of physics of a later day. Perhaps he is most famous for his feat as a philologist in the deciphering of the Rosetta Stone to provide the key for reading Egyptian hieroglyphics, an achievement that he shared with the Frenchman, Champollion. Young was called by Helmholtz the most erudite physician of his generation.

Thomas Hodgkin (1798-1866). Here was another illustrious physician to spring from Quaker stock in or near Yorkshire. He was an active member of the Society of Friends and all his life he wore their plain garb and used the plain language. After studying medicine in Paris and in Edinburgh, he became pathologist, first to Guy's Hospital and later to St. Thomas's Hospital. As pathologist he established his name in medical history by being the first to describe the glandular disease now known as Hodgkin's disease; he was also the first to describe aortic regurgitation. For a while he practiced medicine in London. In addition, Thomas Hodgkin was a philanthropist and a reformer concerned with poor housing and poor sanitation, with alcoholism, with the abuse of children (especially as chimney sweeps), and with slavery (he founded the antislavery organization, the Aborigines Protective Society). He traveled extensively with his friend and fellow philanthropist, Sir Moses Montefiore, and died of dysentery in the Holy Land; he is buried at Jaffa.

Sir Francis Galton (1822-1911). The Galtons were a Quaker family in Birmingham. Francis Galton, a cousin of Charles Darwin, studied medicine at the Birmingham General Hospital and at Kings College Medical School in London. With his medical skill he allied his abilities as mathematician and psychologist to establish the Biometric Laboratory at the University of London; in this capacity he became the founder of the statistics of eugenics, or genetics. He made the very practical discovery of the use of fingerprints for absolute identification. In addition, as a meteorologist he first described anticyclones, and as a geographer he explored Africa. Thus he was a most versatile Fellow of the Royal Society.

Sir Jonathan Hutchinson (1828-1913). This famous Quaker physician came from a Quaker family in Selby in Yorkshire, and his Quakerism was said to be important to him throughout his life. After an apprenticeship under ***Caleb Williams,*** Quaker surgeon and preacher, he studied medicine in York and at St. Bartholomew's Hospital in London. For many years he was chief surgeon to the London Hospital. He also practiced general medicine with special interest in the fields of dermatology, syphilology, and ophthalmology. He was a prolific medical writer and was the first to describe the signs in congenital syphilis of deformed teeth, interstitial keratitis, and deafness ("Hutchinson's triad"), as well as the diseases of temporal arteritis and sarcoidosis. He was a Fellow of the Royal Society, president of the Royal College of Surgeons, and was knighted at the end of his life.

Joseph (Lord) Lister (1827-1912). Joseph Lister, perhaps the most eminent figure in British medicine in the 19th century, can be claimed for Quaker medicine only by virtue of his birth and upbringing. He was born and reared in a Quaker family in Essex.

(They lived next door to the famous garden in Upton that had been created by Dr. John Fothergill.) But as a young man he married the daughter of James Syme, his surgical chief in Edinburgh, and thus, having married out of meeting, he lost his membership in the Society of Friends. Nevertheless, he adhered to Quaker beliefs all his life and is surely a major contributor to the Quaker heritage in medicine.

Lister was educated at University College Hospital and attained his M.B. and F.R.C.S. in 1852. Following his surgical training under Syme in Edinburgh, he became professor of surgery at, progressively, Glasgow, Edinburgh, and, in his later years, Kings College in London. His great achievement, of course, was the discovery and development of surgical antisepsis. His demonstration that the sepsis of surgical operative fields could be prevented revolutionized the tables of surgical mortality and became, along with the discovery of anesthesia, the cornerstone of modern surgery as we know it. Lister spent a major portion of his professional life trying to persuade his surgical colleagues, often against much opposition, to make use of his discovery. He became a friend of Pasteur and established an institute in England to provide vaccinations against rabies.

Joseph Lister served in turn as president of the Royal Society, the Royal College of Surgeons, and the British Association for the Advancement of Science; he was the first medical man to be elevated to the House of Lords. Yet throughout his busy life, filled both with honors and with controversies, he retained a gentle and sweet character that demonstrated his religious faith and benefited his patients. In a letter written to his sister Jane in 1857 he said:

> I trust I may be enabled in the treatment of patients always to act with a single eye to their good and therefore to the glory of our Heavenly Father. If a man be able to act in this spirit, and is favoured to feel something of the sustaining love of God in his work, truly the practice of surgery is a glorious occupation.

Comment

These five "Quaker" doctors exemplified the application of well-educated, inquiring minds to the development of medical science in the mid-19th century. These men also were concerned for their patients, an attribute undoubtedly shared with a host of other physicians and surgeons, Quaker and non-Quaker, of their century. They showed less direct interest, with the exception of Thomas Hodgkin, in the social reforms being undertaken at that time by the Society of Friends, such as the abolition of slavery (Joseph Sturge) and prison reform (Elizabeth Fry). Nevertheless, their major roles in the advances of medical and surgical practices contributed to the welfare of countless patients, and as such they are a proud part of the Quaker medical heritage.

Latter Nineteenth and Early Twentieth Centuries

The Rise of Quaker Evangelism and Foreign Missions

AT THE END of the last century the Society of Friends began to reach out both at home and abroad with their Christian message. The Friends Foreign Mission Association (FFMA) was created. The modern era of Quaker committees and organized programs began. Although Quaker doctors were closely involved in these new activities, the medical heritage of Friends is still best told in terms of individual medical men and, now, women.

Doctors in Foreign Missions

William Wilson (1857-1909). Here perhaps is the first Quaker medical missionary. As a very young man William Wilson taught at Waterford School in Ireland and there joined Friends. At the age of 20 he felt called to serve as a missionary in Madagascar and was sent out in 1877 under the auspices of the Friends Foreign Missionary Association. In Madagascar he set up schools for the natives under primitive conditions, but soon realized that one of their greatest needs was medical care. To meet this need he undertook on his first furlough in 1880 a year's study at the London Hospital. On his second furlough, although he was married and had a family, he was allowed four years' leave of absence to complete, in 1890, his qualifications as M.R.C.S. and L.R.C.P. He had already started one small hospital in a country district, and on his return to Madagascar in 1894 he took charge of a new hospital that had been opened by Queen Ranavalona III in 1891 in the capital, Antananarivo. He had a special interest in the training of Malagasy medical students and nurses. In 1895 Madagascar was occupied by French forces and a year later the hospital was requisitioned; Dr. Wilson subsequently moved to one of the outlying districts. On his third furlough in 1900 he accompanied Watson Grace, the general secretary of the FFMA, on a deputation to what was then the Friends Syrian Mission, where medical work also was opening up. Watson Grace contracted typhoid from which he died, and in 1901 William Wilson was deemed to be the person to succeed him as general secretary of the FFMA. He served in this capacity, traveling widely in China, India, Syria, and Ceylon, until his death in 1909. "He was," said Sir George Newman, "a strong, practical man, loving and beloved, and clothed in shining armour."

Henry T. Hodgkin (1877-1933). Henry Hodgkin came from an evangelical Quaker family in Darlington, County Durham. After attending Leighton Park School and Cambridge, he trained at St. Thomas's and received his M.B. in 1902. In 1904 Dr. Hodgkin entered the mission field and went out to China. In Chengtu in West China his medical work was combined with teaching and preaching and he became primarily a missionary statesman. In 1910 he was recalled to become secretary of the FFMA in succession to Dr. William Wilson. During his ten years in this post he wrote a textbook on medical missions and became an ardent pacifist during the First World War, helping to found the Fellowship of Reconciliation. In 1920 he revisited China and from 1923 to 1929, during the difficult period of civil war, he served as secretary of the National Christian Council of China. Finally, from 1930 to the time of his death in 1933, Henry Hodgkin, as the first director, worked hard to launch Pendle Hill School, the new Quaker center for religious studies near Philadelphia. Pendle Hill owes much of its early success to Henry Hodgkin, whose warm personality and deep religious faith had won him a tremendous circle of friends the world over.

Lucy E. Harris (1873-1962). The Quaker mission to the province of Szechwan in West China began in the last decade of the 19th century under the leadership of Robert Davidson, Isaac Mason, and others. But not until 1899, five years before the arrival of Henry Hodgkin, did a medically qualified Quaker join the mission. This was Lucy E. Harris, a young woman Friend who gained her M.B. at the Royal Free Hospital in London that year. Her medical work in Szechwan was especially notable for her obstetrical work, for the Friends Hospital and School for Nurses that she established in the town of Tungchwan, and for her dedication to her Chinese patients. Dr. Harris gave 46 years of her life to her medical work in China in a career that included a series of adventurous encounters with bandits and soldiers during many years of civil and foreign wars. Only after the end of World War II did "this dauntless little woman" consent to retire from China and return to her homeland.

W. Henry Davidson (1872-1958). The second medical doctor to join the Friends mission group in West China was Dr. Henry Davidson, who went out in 1901 and joined Dr. Lucy Harris in Tungchwan. Henry Davidson was one of the four Davidson brothers who served many years as Friends missionaries in China. The oldest brother, Robert, was the pioneer in 1886; and the other brothers, Adam and Henry and Alfred, followed in 1897 and 1901. Their father, Adam Davidson, had been a British soldier who in 1860 had witnessed the sack of the emperor's summer palace outside Peking. This so distressed him that he obtained his release from the army, returned home, and joined the Society of Friends in Ireland. His concern to redress the wrong done to China eventually led to the missionary service of his four sons and later of one grandson. In 1903 Dr. Henry Davidson married Laura Morris, a nurse, and subsequently built and headed the mission hospital in Suining. During the revolution of 1911-1912 he cared for the wounded in Hankow. In 1939 he returned to England to Selly Oak where he served as an elder of Bournville Meeting.

William Warder Cadbury (1877-1959). The major American medical worker in the Friends mission field in China was Dr. William Cadbury. A member of the Quaker family of Cadburys in Philadelphia (Henry J. Cadbury was one of his brothers, and Rufus Jones became his brother-in-law), William Cadbury graduated from Haverford College and the University of Pennsylvania School of Medicine. In 1910 he went out to China and served in Lingnan University in Canton where he became professor of medicine. In 1943 he was interned by the Japanese and then returned to Philadelphia. He went back to Canton for three years, 1946 to 1949, before retiring. William Cadbury was never reconciled to the Communist takeover of China, but in 1955 he wrote: "It is consoling that all has not been annihilated as was the custom of the earlier conquerors of the world."

Practitioners at Home

Ann E. Clark (1844-1924). Dr. Clark was the first woman in the Society of Friends to qualify in medicine in Great Britain. A member of the Quaker family of Clarks in Street, Somerset, she determined in her late twenties to study medicine. At that time no women were admitted to medical schools in England. However, Edinburgh decided to try admitting a small group of women into the medical school; Ann Clark was one of them. Part way through training, the university changed its policy and as a result Ann Clark transferred to the University of Berne, Switzerland, where she received her M.D. in 1877. After taking her M.R.C.P. in Dublin and undertaking special studies in Paris, Vienna, and Boston, she went to Birmingham where she spent the rest of her professional life. She served as a surgeon at the Midland Hospital for Women and the Childrens Hospital and was associated with Lawson Tait in pioneer work in abdominal and gynecological surgery. In addition she had a large medical practice in which she was much beloved as "Dr. Annie." She was a regular attendant at Bull St. Meeting and was a life-long member of the Society of Friends.

Mary D. Sturge (1862-1925). Here was another early woman doctor in Birmingham. A member in that city of the Quaker families Sturge and Lloyd, Mary Sturge received her M.B. from London University in 1891 and practiced in Birmingham until her death in 1925. Her greatest social interest was in the cause of temperance, and she was coauthor with Victor Horsley of the book *Alcohol and the Human Body*. In 1920, at the end of the First World War, she directed the program for famine relief of children in the northern Tyrol.

R. Hingston Fox (1853-1924). This name brings to our attention what surely is the most extensive medical family in English Quakerdom, the Fox family of Falmouth. ***Joseph Fox*** (1729-1785), Quaker surgeon of Falmouth, was the ancestor and the first of some 21 doctors and three pharmacists in seven generations of this remarkable Quaker family (not counting those doctors and nurses who descended through the female lines). One of his three medical sons was ***Edward Long Fox*** (1761-1835), M.D. Edinburgh, who founded near Bristol the first Quaker asylum for the mentally ill in England (see Part I). In the fourth generation of the family there were six brothers, four of whom were physicians or surgeons and one a pharmacist. The eldest of these brothers, ***Joseph John Fox*** (1821-1897), M.R.C.S., of Stoke Newington, had six sons, five of whom were doctors and who constituted the fifth medical generation in the Fox family.

Dr. Hingston Fox was one of these five medical brothers. After training at the London Hospital (M.R.C.S. 1874, M.D. and M.R.C.P. 1884, and later F.R.C.P.), he went into general practice in Finsbury Park, London; in 1902 he established a very busy general consulting practice on Harley Street. He was a man of wide interests: he wrote two medical biographies, one of William Hunter and one of John Fothergill; he translated Greek texts; and he cultivated his hobbies of antiquities, ornithology, and botany. He was a life-long member and active minister of the Society of Friends and was much involved in Quaker activities. These included the Friends Foreign Mission Association for whom he visited the Friends Mission in Syria, and the Council for International Service which involved him in relief work in Germany after the First World War. He was the author of *The Quaker Touch,* the message that went with that aid.

Robert Fortescue Fox (1858-1940). Fortescue Fox was another of the sons of Dr. Joseph Fox, and he, too, trained at the London Hospital (M.D. and, late in life, F.R.C.P.). At 25, because he was delicate, he started practice in the country in the Scottish village of Strathpeffer, already well known as a spa. As physician there, he was greatly impressed by the usefulness of physical treatment; and when in early middle age he went back to London, he became an authority on British and foreign spas and their methods, described in his book *Medical Hydrology.*

In addition he was urging the revival and development of physical treatment for patients who could never go to spas; and during the First World War he was able, with Robert Jones, to demonstrate its value for disabled soldiers. He insisted that while they were having treatment, patients should also have whatever training or retraining they needed for their future work; and in this he was a pioneer in what was later called *rehabilitation.* "Treatment *and* training," he used to say. After the war his efforts led to the creation of a village settlement at Enham in Hampshire for disabled ex-servicemen, and for a year he was its medical director.

However, his most lasting influence was on the care of rheumatism, and in this field, too, he was a pioneer. In season and out, he preached his message that far too little was being done for the vast number of people with arthritis who could be helped by physical treatment. Very slowly this truth was accepted, partly through the work of the International League against Rheumatism and partly through the Empire Rheumatism Council, both of which he helped to found.

Fortescue Fox was also a practical internationalist. Like others of his family, he was for many years the London chairman of the Lebanon Hospital for Mental Diseases at Asfuriyeh, near Beirut; much of his later life was spent on his particular offspring, the International Society of Hydrology. He was indeed a Friend of wide medical and social concerns.

E. Claude Taylor (1871-1924). Claude Taylor came from a Quaker family in London and was a second cousin of Joseph Lister. He qualified at Guy's Hospital in 1894 (M.D. 1895, F.R.C.S. 1896, and M.S. in surgery in 1897 at University of London). His professional life was spent in general practice and surgery in London's Hampstead. He was assistant medical officer to the London Temperance Hospital, attended in the Bunhill Medical Mission in East London, and was medical officer to the Hampstead Infirmary. He had a wide practice among devoted patients who included Ramsay MacDonald, subsequently the first Labour prime minister. Dr. Taylor served two terms as a Labour member of the Local Burough Council. His social welfare work included teaching the adult school and lecturing widely on temperance. He was an active member of the Society of Friends and was one of the principal founders of Hampstead Meeting. During World War I he took a strong stand as a pacifist but was allowed to serve as a civilian surgeon when the Hampstead Infirmary was taken over as a military hospital; he strongly supported other conscientious objectors. Shortly after the war he died of leukemia at the age of 53. Of him Sir George Newman said, "He was a disciple of Hippocrates and a disciple of George Fox . . . for one and a same reason, there is a divine power which alone lifts a man to the highest."

Claude Taylor fathered another medical Quaker family: two of his four sons were Quaker doctors. ***Robert Taylor*** was a surgeon in Hertfordshire before his retirement, and ***A. Brian Taylor***, late physician in Birmingham, was an expert on diseases of the chest and a pioneer in cardiac pacemaking. Another son, Christopher Taylor, while not a medico, was treasurer for many years of the Friends Service Council which conducted many relief programs abroad. Clare Norton, nurse and health visitor, a daughter of Christopher Taylor and thus a granddaughter of Claude Taylor and, incidentally, through her mother, a great-granddaughter of William Wilson, is carrying on the family tradition. She served with the Quaker Service Team in Algeria and for a short time at Brummana High School in Lebanon. More recently, she worked on the Home Care Service of the St. Josephs Hospice, Hackney,

London. This is part of the movement for the care of the dying in which another Quaker, Dr. Richard Lamerton, is prominent.

Comment

In this group of Quaker doctors we see the evangelical missionary zeal combined with the practical work of medicine, the emergence of the movement for the equality of women with men in medicine, the beginning of organized foreign relief on a large scale, and again the vigorous pursuit of social as well as scientific concerns by active medical practitioners.

Twentieth Century

World Wars I and II and Beyond

OUR PRESENT CENTURY is characterized by the tremendous growth of science and technology, including that in the field of medicine, and by violent conflicts and social and political upheavals. These modern challenges to Quakerism led to the rapid growth of alternative services for conscientious objectors to military participation; to the rapid expansion of large-scale programs for the relief of afflicted peoples and destitute refugees of whatever race, creed, or political allegiance; and to renewed search for spiritual, as well as physical, resources for human life. To these endeavors doctors in the Society contributed, as they did to the growth of medical science and its application to human needs.

A Pioneer in Public Health

Sir George Newman (1870-1948). And so we come to one of the outstanding Quaker medical personalities, some of whose dicta concerning his fellow Quaker doctors have already been quoted. George Newman, son of Henry S. Newman, who was editor of the *Friend* and one of the founders of the FFMA, trained in medicine at Edinburgh and became a distinguished public-health officer in London. A great believer in preventive medicine, he served as district health officer in Finsbury where he studied the effect of overcrowding on infant mortality and set up a series of baby clinics; he was knighted in 1911. When the Ministry of Health was established in 1919, Sir George became its first Chief Medical Officer. In this capacity he initiated the National Maternity and Child Welfare Service, based on his experience in Finsbury. He wrote the key postwar report on the reorganization of British medical education and was instrumental in establishing the Postgraduate Medical School and the London School of Hygiene and Tropical Medicine. He was also active in the movement for the education of working men; he was the driving force in the Westminster Men's Adult School and was a member of the National Adult School Council.

George Newman functioned in the center of British Quakerism as editor of the *Friends Quarterly Examiner* for 40 years. He wrote extensively as an essayist in the fields of Quaker history and biography as well as in the history of medicine. He and Arnold Rowntree, Quaker industrialist from York, were close friends and supporters of Rufus Jones and William Charles Braithwaite as the two latter completed their monumental history of Quakerism begun with John Wilhelm Rowntree. During World War I George Newman was a prime mover in setting up the Friends' Ambulance Unit (FAU) and served as chairman of its council throughout the war. Again, during World War II when the FAU was reactivated and expanded, he gave it his advice and close support. George Newman keenly propounded as "cardinal tenets of Quakerism" the principle of the "Inward Light" and reliance on spiritual experience in a noninstitutionalized way of life. In words that are as true now as they were when he wrote them in 1946 near the end of his life, he asked,

> Has the world no need of Quakerism today? Amid its wealth and poverty, its strife and ostentation, its growing complexity, its waywardness, its wilfullness, its love of self, its lust and sin, its seeking for a sign, is there still no place, still a glorious call for those who belong to the family of the Children of Light?

Great Physiologist

Sir Joseph Barcroft (1872-1947). Joseph Barcroft was born into an old Quaker family of linen manufacturers in Ulster. His interest in science and natural history was developed first at Bootham School in York. In 1896 he received his B.A. from Cambridge and after a few months of medical studies decided on a career of full-time physiology at Cambridge. Because of his great contributions to medical science in this field, he is included in this survey. In 1925 he became professor of physiology at Cambridge, and until the time of his death he was a world figure. His scientific contributions included analyses of respiration and mountain sickness at high altitudes (studied especially in the Peruvian Andes), oxygen therapy to gassed soldiers, the basic physiology of hemoglobin, and the dynamics of blood circulation in the pregnant mother and in the fetus. He was knighted in 1935.

In 1900 Joseph Barcroft visited the Doukhobors who were newly settled in Canada, and subsequently he served on the Doukhobor Committee of London Yearly Meeting. He was a regular attendant of Friends Meeting until the First World War; thereafter he was a nominal member of the Society. But his Quaker upbringing and beliefs did much to mold him into the genial, warm-hearted, open-minded man and scientist that he was.

Quaker Relief Projects and Doctors in World War I

The onset of the First World War in 1914 posed a tremendous challenge to the Society of Friends in Great Britain. Beyond supporting those individuals who suffered for their conscientious refusal of military service, the Society sought to take positive steps to relieve and help the vast numbers of victims of the war, military and civilian. Two organizations were set up: the Friends Ambulance Unit, headed by Sir George Newman, and the Friends War Victims Relief Committee (FWVRC), whose name was taken from the committee that had existed during the Franco-Prussian War in 1870-1871. The history of the activities of these two Quaker organizations during World War I and the succeeding decade, especially in Russia, has been set forth in detail elsewhere (see references); it is pertinent in this paper only to indicate the nature of the medical work undertaken and some of the Quaker personnel who, under such difficult circumstances, contributed to the Quaker heritage in medicine.

In the Friends Ambulance Unit in the First World War there were relatively few qualified Quaker doctors; the lay members of the unit who were sent to France in the early years of the war functioned primarily as ambulance drivers and hospital orderlies working with Allied military medical units. Other young Quakers worked to help the civilian populations in the devastated battle areas and some of the help was medical. One of the best-known examples was the maternity hospital established at Chalons-sur-Marne in 1914 and directed for five years by Dr. ***Hilda Clark*** and Edith Pye. One of the young FAU members was ***John Rosslyn Earp***, who subsequently studied medicine and became an influential administrator and educator in public health in the United States, first in New Mexico and later in the state of New York. During his professional life he was severely handicapped by, and died prematurely of, the tuberculosis that he had contracted while working as a young English Quaker among French civilians behind the lines. Several of the FAU members who were doctors moved on to Russia in 1916 when the FWVRC started programs in the Volga basin for relief of war refugees from Poland and western Russia. Centers for food distribution and homes for children were set up, and a number of small hospitals were established or reactivated. The medical problems were myriad: typhoid, poliomyelitis, typhus, dysentery, measles, scarlet fever, diphtheria, whooping cough, smallpox, malaria, tuberculosis, trachoma. The medical personnel of the first relief party from England included Drs. John Rickman, Tylor Fox, George Pearson, and Herbert Manning, as well as nurses Ellen Bull, Elsie Fox, Theodora Williams, and May Pattison; the lay members included Florence Barrow, Jack Catchpool, Robert Tatlock, and Theodore Rigg. In the following summer of 1917 the party was joined by six young Quaker women sent by the American Friends Service Committee; although they were social workers and not nurses, they were quickly pressed into nursing duties. In 1918 the whole party was caught up in the turmoil of the Russian Revolution and was forced to withdraw across Siberia working with the hordes of refugees as they went.

Of these Quaker medical workers in Russia we may note especially Drs. John Rickman and Tylor Fox. John Rickman (1891-1951) headed the hospital in Mogolova and initiated a policy of insisting that the relatives of patients should learn to do the active nursing. Of this relief program in Russia during 1916 to 1918, he wrote, "We came out to Russia filled with the idea of doing only 'emergency' work, but in addition we found work of even greater importance. By keeping open a few of their hospitals we are sustaining the people in their growing belief in the efficacy of self-help." In after years in England Rickman practiced psychiatry and psychoanalysis. ***J. Tylor Fox*** (1885-1949) was the son of Dr. R. Hingston Fox and thus was one of the sixth generation of the Fox medical family. After the war he became a student of epilepsy and directed the Lingfield Colony for epileptics. He was an active member of the Society of Friends. His son, Dr. Richard Fox, is a psychiatrist and an active member of the Samaritans, the organization for aiding would-be suicides.

Quaker relief and medical efforts in postwar Russia did not end with the withdrawal of the first FWVRC and AFSC workers across Siberia. In the new Soviet nation famine was widespread and Quaker workers returned in 1920. Of these, two were from the original AFSC group who had come first in 1917: ***Nancy Babb*** went on to found a maternity hospital in Totskoye in 1923; ***Anna Haines*** became an instructor in a new nurses training hospital in Moscow and planned a new center which was taken over by the Russians in 1926. The English group included ***Dr. Melville McKenzie***, who was trained in public health. In Buzuluk he established certain measures such as delousing to prevent epidemics, and set up a lab for the diagnosis and treatment of malaria. Another Quaker doctor in public health in Russia during the early years of the Soviet regime was ***Harry Timbres.*** Harry and Rebecca Timbres, who had met as American Quaker relief workers in Poland in 1921, returned to

Russia with their two daughters in 1936; in the interim he had trained in medicine at Johns Hopkins and the London School of Tropical Medicine and worked in malaria control in India from 1929 to 1935. In Russia Dr. Timbres and his family were sent to a new town in the Maruski Republic on the Volga where he set up a research center for the eradication of malaria. In May 1937 Harry Timbres caught typhus and died. Rebecca Timbres has written a moving account of their story in the book *We Didn't Ask Utopia.* Quaker medicine brought sacrifice as well as accomplishment.

Practitioners on the Home Front

Of the many British Quaker doctors who were active at home during the major portion of this century spanning the two world wars, two may be mentioned as exemplars of the spirit of Quakerism in medicine.

Henry T. Gillett (1870-1955). Dr. Gillett for many years practiced medicine in Oxford. There he fostered the Friends Meeting ("Father of the Meeting") and traveled widely in the ministry. It was his concern that led to the establishment in 1950 of Charney Manor for small religious retreats. He served as chairman of the Home Service Committee of London Yearly Meeting. In the Oxford community he was active on behalf of the adult school, temperance, and peace movements. He was a city councillor for many terms and was mayor of Oxford in 1938-1939. He wrote several books, including *The Spiritual Basis of Democracy,* published in 1952.

Howard E. Collier (1890-1953). Dr. Collier was a general practitioner in Redditch and area medical health officer, as well as a lecturer in industrial hygiene at the University of Birmingham. He had joined the Society of Friends after the First World War and became deeply convinced of the need to heal the spiritual, as well as the physical and mental, ills of his patients. He has been a prime Quaker advocate of spiritual healing in our modern era (see below).

In addition to these two physicians, the Quaker heritage in medicine has been upheld and contributed to by a host of unsung Quaker clinicians—general practitioners and consultants, physicians and surgeons, nurses and paramedical workers—who, although unnamed here, must not be forgotten.

Medical Scientists, Teachers, and Editors

In the same period spanning the two world wars, Quaker physicians continued to contribute to medical science and learning; a few of the outstanding contributors follow.

W. Russell (Lord) Brain (1895-1966). Born into a non-Quaker family in Reading, Russell Brain read law at Oxford before the First World War. In 1915 he joined the Friends Ambulance Unit where he became an X-ray technologist. After the war he taught psychology at Oxford, and studied medicine and then neurology, first under Sir Charles Sherrington and then under Sir Henry Head in London. His career as a neurologist was a distinguished one, and he wrote a major textbook on the subject. Knighted in 1952, Sir Russell Brain served as president of the Royal College of Physicians of London from 1950 to 1957, and of the British Association; subsequently he was elevated to the House of Lords. In 1963 he chaired the so-called Brain Committee on Drug Addiction. A Fellow of the Royal Society, he wrote widely on subjects in many fields beyond his major interest in medicine and psychology. A physician-philosopher indeed!

Russell Brain and his wife Stella joined the Society of Friends in the 1930s and were members first of Kingston and then of Wimbledon meetings. He was a quiet , reserved man, but his aloofness was deceptive for he had a warm home life and a sense of fun. In 1944 he gave the Swarthmore Lecture on the subject, "Man, Society, and Religion," in which he stated his belief that Quakers tend to underestimate the importance of thought in religious life, and that Quakerism offers a bridge between life of the mind and life of matter, between religion and modern scientific culture, that "for Quakerism life is a sacrament . . . we dwell at the intersection of time and eternity and we are called to realize in time values which are eternal."[3]

3. In light comment on Russell Brain's theme in his Swarthmore Lecture,

Cuthbert E. Dukes (1890-1977). Cuthbert Dukes was born in Somerset, the son of a Congregational minister, and trained in medicine at Edinburgh (M.B. in 1914). He served in the R.A.M.C. during the First World War; subsequently he became a prominent clinical pathologist in London and an authority on tumors of the rectum, colon, and genitourinary tract. He was an Honorary Fellow of the Royal Society of Medicine, president of the Medical Society of London and of the Association of Clinical Pathologists.

Dr. Cuthbert Dukes and his wife, Dr. Ethel Dukes, a child psychologist, joined Friends in 1924 after he had become a convinced pacifist. They were members of Westminister Meeting where he served as clerk and as president of the Mens Adult School. Subsequently they moved to Wimbledon Meeting where they were close friends of Russell and Stella Brain. Dr. Dukes was active in the Friends Fellowship of Healing. He was a kindly, unassuming man with a whimsical sense of humor in addition to "his gentleness compounded of an inner tranquility and wisdom which was strongly influenced by his Quaker faith."

Lionel S. Penrose (1899-1972). Dr. Penrose was a leading specialist in the field of mental retardation and human genetics and was particularly renowned for his studies of Down's syndrome. He served as professor of eugenics (later human genetics) at University College, London, from 1945 to 1965 and as director of the Kennedy-Galton Centre in St. Albans. from 1965 until his death. He became a Fellow of the Royal Society in 1953.

Lionel Penrose was an extremely versatile man as an artist, a musician, a chess player, a mathematician, and an inventor of "self-reproducing objects." He was of a Quaker family, and his father, J. Doyle Penrose, was the artist who painted what is probably the most famous picture of a Friend's meeting, *The Presence in the Midst.* Dr. Penrose was a member of Colchester

---

William Hughes of the Yearly Meeting wrote:

> If we give thought no proper part,
> Then semi-Quakers we remain,
> Besides a trembling of the heart,
> We need a rustle of the brain.

Meeting. He advocated scientific study of social behavior to eliminate war, was active in the Medical Association for the Prevention of War, and was treasurer of War Resisters International.

Egbert C. Morland (1875-1955). Born in Croydon and educated at Bootham School in York, Egbert Morland trained in medicine at St. Bartholomew's (M.B. in 1898). Because he contracted tuberculosis, he spent ten years in Switzerland where, in Arosa, he became a specialist in the treatment of the disease. During World War I he did relief work on the Marne and afterwards he joined the editorial staff of *The Lancet*, where he was editor from 1937 until his retirement to Yorkshire in 1944. During his life in London he served on the Sibford School Committee and attended regularly Friends House Meeting. He was a father-figure to many Quaker doctors and medical students.

Sir Theodore Fox (1899-). Here we have another Quaker doctor who became one of this century's great medical editors. T. F. Fox is the son of Robert Fortescue Fox and hence is another member of the sixth generation of the medical Fox family. He attended Leighton Park School, served with the FAU in France, and went to Cambridge. Apart from three years in the R.A.M.C., his professional life from 1939 was all spent on the editorial staff of *The Lancet*—for the last 20 years as editor, succeeding Egbert Morland. In his Heath Clark Lectures of 1963, "Crisis in Communication: The Function and Future of Medical Journals," he gave a cogent analysis of the problem of multiplication of medical articles and journals. His son, Dr. Robin Fox, as present deputy editor of *The Lancet* will continue to wrestle with these problems.

"Robbie" Fox, as he is called by his friends, although not an active Quaker, has been a life-long member of the Society of Friends from which he has derived his ethical values. The Quaker concern for the whole man is reflected in his Harveian Oration to the Royal College of Physicians in 1965 on "The Purposes of Medicine":

> With all its faults the profession to which we belong is not a body of technologists interested solely in the means by which physical or

> mental processes can be restored to normal; it is a body of doctors seeking to use these means to an end—to help patients to cope with their lives. . . . The doctor has learned more about disease, and must go on learning; but he is, and must always be, a human being devoted first to human beings.

Donald Court (1912-). Professor Court is a pediatrician and a university teacher. From 1955 to 1972 he held the James Spence Chair of Child Health at the University of Newcastle upon Tyne and through long-term family studies developed the social and educational aspects of pediatrics. In 1973 he became president of the British Paediatric Association and was appointed chairman of a special government committee to review child-health services in England and Wales; the committee report, "Fit for the Future," was released at the end of 1976 and calls for widespread and long-term reorganization of continuing therapeutic and preventive care of children.

Influenced by a long friendship with Dr. Howard Collier, Donald Court joined Friends in 1934 while a medical student in Birmingham. He remains an active Friend, an elder first of Newcastle upon Tyne, and now of Bradford-on-Avon Meeting, and is a trustee of the Joseph Rowntree Charitable Trust. In an article in *The Friend* in 1965 entitled "A Scientific Age and a Declining Church; What Has a Friend to Say?" he gave a compelling account of his personal reconciliation of his scientific beliefs as a physician and his religious beliefs as a Christian and a Friend. In part he said:

> For me worship is a rational response; but reverence for the universe, for life and for man needs constant reinforcement. . . . I find this in Meeting for Worship and I could not do without it. Worship in silence is right for me, because as a doctor and a teacher I have special need for silence. . . . Friends doctrine is derived from experience and must be consistent with it. We know that actions speak louder than words, and that we must each invest our humanity in practical service; and, as we are part of one another in a deeper sense than we understand, we must be concerned with social justice and community care. In the last analysis I am a Quaker because Friends will never let me forget that real growth is growth in caring.

On the other side of the Atlantic many American clinicians, medical teachers, and medical scientists also were contributing to the Quaker heritage of the 20th century. For these many, two persons will have to stand in this paper.

Joseph Stokes, Jr. (1896-1972). Here again we have a pediatrician and beloved physician to children who was one of the great figures of American medicine and perhaps the outstanding Quaker doctor of his day. The Stokes were another medical family in the Society of Friends. Joseph, Jr., and his brother Dr. ***S. Emlen Stokes,*** sons of Dr. ***Joseph Stokes, Sr.,*** were members of the fifth, and Dr. ***Joseph Stokes III,*** of the sixth generation of this family of Quaker doctors.

The career of Joseph Stokes, Jr., lay in academic pediatrics. His main professional goal was to promote the health of children, and his many young patients—and their parents—were devoted to him. He was William H. Bennett Professor of Pediatrics at the University of Pennsylvania and physician-in-chief to the Childrens Hospital of Philadelphia from 1939 to 1963. During this period he was primarily responsible for developing the Childrens Hospital into one of the great pediatric teaching and research centers of the world. His major scientific contributions were in the field of immunization against infectious diseases: he pioneered the use of gamma globulin as a protection against poliomyelitis and viral hepatitis and, with his collaborators, played a major role in the development of vaccines against influenza, measles, mumps, and rubella. As a member of the Army Epidemiological Board during World War II, he introduced the use of gamma globulin for the prevention of epidemic hepatitis among American troops, and for his dangerous medical missions in the Mediterranean theater of war he received the Medal of Freedom.

Beyond his scientific achievements, Joseph Stokes was a dedicated and liberal humanitarian. He was a great educator and a proponent of comprehensive health care as a right for all. Few civic programs for the improvement of Philadelphia failed to have his active support. During the First World War he was a conscientious objector to military service. During and after the Second World War he served the American Friends Service Committee in multiple capacities in the effort to bring practical services of reconciliation into many areas of conflict: in 1940, relief for children in unoccupied France; in 1958, a mission with two other Quaker doctors (***George Perera*** and ***Samuel Corson***) to Soviet Russia to make medical contacts in the midst of the cold war; more recently, relief to Biafra, to South and North Vietnam, to Bangladesh. As chairman of the Family Planning Committee of the AFSC, he was a key member of the working party that from 1966 to 1970 prepared the book *Who Shall Live? Man's Control over Birth and Death*; and he was a leader of the Friends Medical Society.

Joseph Stokes, Jr., was a friendly, handsome, warm-hearted man, with a close-knit, loving family life. He was a deeply religious man and was devoted to the Society of Friends. In a memorandum that he wrote for his fellow members of the working party who were preparing the book *Who Shall Live?* he said:

> Death is a sacrifice that is biologically necessary to any adequate ethical system in the higher forms of life. This sacrificial motive is emphasized in the Judeo-Christian ethic of the Second Commandment "Love thy neighbor as thyself." . . . As Christ put it man must lose his life in order to find it. Christ accomplished this in his dramatic life and death, and was resurrected in the form of a religious philosophy that is both biologically and theologically timeless in quality. Each person in a small way may accomplish this according to his vision, his capabilities, and his dedication in adding his seemingly minute contribution—a mere drop in the ocean of light flowing over the ocean of darkness, as prophesied by George Fox. . . . Do not the answers to the dilemmas posed by modern science require the recognition that love—in the largest sense—and all the consequences that flow from it is a necessary ingredient of the whole man and the abundant life?

Jonathan E. Rhoads (1907-). Here in another Philadelphia family we have one of the outstanding surgeons of the present day, **Dr. Jonathan Rhoads. His father, Dr. *Edward Rhoads,*** practiced in Germantown; Jonathan married Dr. Teresa Folin (daughter of the pioneer Harvard biochemist Otto Folin) and a number of their sons are in medicine and hospital administration. A graduate of Johns Hopkins Medical School, Jonathan Rhoads has spent his professional career at the University of Pennsylvania where he is surgeon, teacher, and investigator in the surgical sciences. As John Rhea Barton Professor of Surgery, he was chairman of the Department of Surgery and for several years served as provost of the university. As a medical statesman, he has held many important academic and professional positions on local and national levels, including the presidencies of the College of Physicians of Philadelphia, the American College of Surgeons, the American Cancer Society, and the American Philosophical Society. He is prominent in civic affairs and received the Philadelphia Award for 1976.

Jonathan Rhoads is an active member of Philadelphia Yearly Meeting. He has been deeply involved in Quaker education as a trustee of Bryn Mawr College and as chairman of the board of Haverford College. He has assisted the American Friends Service Committee in various relief programs including travel to North Vietnam with medical and surgical supplies for that war-torn area. He, too, has been a leader in the Friends Medical Society and organized the Friends Medical Foundation to give it financial support. In this present-day Quaker "man for all seasons" the Quaker heritage in medicine is well exemplified.

Quaker Medical Projects in World War II and After

Friends Ambulance Unit. With the onset of the Second World War in 1939, the FAU was reactivated. In contrast to its mode of function in World War I, the FAU sent out many more qualified medical members and mounted a wide variety of direct medical services, including local hospitals, dispensaries, public-health programs, as well as the transportation of medical supplies. These medical activities were an integral part of the FAU's worldwide efforts to help the victims of the war and eventually involved more than a thousand professional and lay members, part of whom were young Quakers. The complex and fascinating story of the FAU cannot be told here (for that see A. Tegla Davies's book in the references); it must suffice to indicate the main areas of the above-listed activities of the FAU and the names of some of the medical personnel who were involved.

Finland, 1939: Dr. John Gillespie.

Ethiopia, 1942-1945: Drs. Michael Vaizy, Anthony Husband, Ken Llewellyn, Pat Griffin, John Salter, Alastair McLeish, John Wyon.

China, 1941-1946:

Burma and the retreat: Drs. Robert McClure, surgeon from Canada; Harry Louderbough, an American; Handley Laycock.

Kunming and Chungking: Drs. Quentin Boyd, who died in 1944; Terry Darling; Will Jenkins.

West and Northwest China: Sixteen international medical teams that included British Drs. Andy Brand and Eric Warrington and American Drs. John Perry, Arthur Barr, Ernest Evans, Alan Longshore, and many others, especially nurses.

Greek Islands: Dr. Peter Early.

In Britain many FAU members manned hospital services in blitzed zones and likewise in Germany after the war.

This list can give little inkling of the character and dedication of the members of the Friends Ambulance Unit that lie behind the names of persons and places, but surely they are part of the Quaker heritage in medicine. And not a few of the Quaker and like-minded young lay members came home to study medicine and, as general practitioners in the new National Health Service, to continue serving their fellow men (as, for example, Dr. Edward Cadbury in Shropshire, Dr. Raymond Birkett in Herefordshire, and Dr. Wilfred Dally in Scotland). Finally, no comment about the history of the FAU would be complete without mention of Dr. Hubert Rutter, a very well known Quaker figure in Birmingham, who unstintedly throughout the war gave first-aid lectures to the lay volunteers as they passed through the FAU training camps.

Friends Service Council and American Friends Service Committee. During and after the end of World War II these two Quaker organizations, separately and together, have carried out many programs that have included medical activities. During the war most American conscientious objectors were not allowed to go overseas, and as a result the AFSC organized and administered the Civilian Public Service (CPS) to provide an alternative to military service. Many young Quakers and other CPS members worked long and hard as orderlies in institutions for the mentally ill. Some of the CPS men volunteered for the dangerous role of experimental subjects for critical research on new drugs for the treatment of malaria and on the nature and transmission of viral hepatitis. After the war, AFSC and FSC medical activities and personnel included the hospital in Kunsan, Korea; Dr. Gordon Barclay and his wife Celia at the Childrens Hospital in Saigon, South Vietnam; Dr. Margery Nelson, Dorothy Weller, physical therapist, and Roger Marshall, prosthetist, at the physiotherapy rehabilitation unit at Quang Ngai; Drs. Jonathan E. Rhoads and George A. Perera, delivery of medical supplies in North Vietnam; Drs. Herbert Bowles, Johan Eliot, and William Lotspeich, active in hospital dispensaries and public-health programs in India, Algeria, Tunisia, Mexico, and West Africa. Organizations other than AFSC and FSC, such as the following, have had the services of Quaker doctors and nurses abroad: Dr. Alex M. Burgess, Jr. (who had been AFSC medical administrator of the CPS during the war), a cardio-vascular epidemiologist in the World Health Organization (WHO) Geneva office; Elfrieda Sollman, R.N., WHO supervisor of public-health nursing in South America; Dr. Frank Catchpool in Lambaréné for a period with Albert Schweitzer; and Dr. Frank Lepreau in charge of the Albert Schweitzer Hospital in Haiti. These names are only some of the dedicated members of the Society of Friends who have given medical service abroad.

In many of the countries receiving Quaker relief the need for family planning pressed the AFSC to try to formulate a Quaker "policy" on contraception and abortion. Quaker physicians such as Dr. Lovett Dewees, gynecologist, of Philadelphia had pioneered providing birth-control clinics, but no Quaker stand on the matter had been formulated as such. Therefore, a working party of Quaker physicians and AFSC staff members was convened, and over a period of three years it thrashed out the ethical and religious issues involved. Joining Henry J. Cadbury, Lorraine Cleveland, Helen Jennings, and Julia and Harry Abrahamson from the AFSC were Drs. John C. Cobb, Elizabeth Conard Corkey, Richard L. Day, Johan W. Eliot, J. Russell Elkinton, and Joseph Stokes, Jr. The results of their deliberations were published in 1970 in the book *Who Shall Live? Man's Control over Birth and Death.* In the final chapter on "Some Answers for Today" the tentative conclusions of the working party included the following statements:

> We believe that the population crisis is so threatening to the quality of human life that for the sake of the individual, the family, and society, we must bring population and resources into balance by learning to control our fertility. Toward this end, we believe that contraception is by far preferable to abortion. But we also believe that abortion, performed under proper conditions, is preferable to the birth of an unwanted child. . . .
>
> We believe that married couples should have the benefit of the best medical and genetic counseling obtainable when genetic or congenital difficulties are anticipated in their children. . . . We are opposed to compulsory abortion or to compulsory sterilization. . . . Direct genetic manipulation to improve the breeding of men seems to us to be socially and morally undesirable as well as scientifically impractical. . . .
>
> We approve withholding therapy or withdrawing the supportive therapy that is keeping an unconscious person alive if, by evidence of brain death or such other evidence as the medical profession deems valid, it is the judgment of the medical profession that the patient's brain is irreparably damaged and he will never recover consciousness. . . . We believe that death should be viewed in proper perspective, as a natural part of the process of life.

A similar approach to another ethical problem was carried out in 1963 in England by a group of Quaker psychiatrists, Drs. Richard Fox, Lotti Rosenberg, and Alfred Torrie, and workers for the Friends Home Service Committee and resulted in the publication, *Towards a Quaker View of Sex.* Neither of these efforts spoke for the Society of Friends as a whole but did exemplify the concern of many Friends for the right solution of health problems on a religious and spiritual basis.

Quaker doctors in the 20th century, as well as in the 17th century, have on occasion formed themselves into groups. The ***Quaker Medical Society*** was set up in Great Britain after the First World War but at present is quiescent. The ***Friends Medical Society*** was created by a group of young Quaker doctors who had been conscientious objectors in World War II, under the leadership of Dr. J. Huston Westover. This society has continued to meet at least annually, and its Bicentennial symposium, under the chairmanship of Dr. Victor C. Vaughan III, held in Philadelphia April 9 and 10, 1976, was the occasion for this paper.

Finally, one more Quaker organization in Great Britain should be mentioned, the ***Friends Fellowship of Healing.*** This fellowship, established more than 40 years ago between the world wars, consists of some 46 groups of Friends who in prayer support those who are ill. This spiritual healing, to restore the wholeness of a person at all levels, is sought by the use of intercessary prayer to bring the one in need and the praying group into unity with God. Thus we return full cycle to the spiritual healing of George Fox as we end this survey.

Comment

Thus, in the Quaker doctors and health workers of the 20th century we see the flowering of three characteristics of the Quaker medical heritage: the experimental drive of the inquiring mind, the care for the whole patient (for his spiritual as well as for his physical and mental well-being), and the concern for the improvement of social conditions that lead to better health for greater numbers of people. This latter concern is manifested by the creation of new and larger Quaker service organizations for relief and reconciliation in war areas and in underdeveloped nations.

Concluding Discussion

THIS SURVEY of the history of Quakers in medicine over the three centuries of the existence of the Society of Friends has focused on people rather than on technical achievement and organizations. Such attention is due to the conviction that the Quaker approach to health is implicit in the lives and actions of a host of Quaker doctors and health workers and that it is there that we must look for the contributions of Quakerism to the profession.

Two Quaker Doctors Speak on Quakerism and Medicine

Occasionally medical members of the Society of Friends do speak explicitly on the relation of their religion to their profession of medicine. Two of the 20th century doctors discussed above may be quoted.

Dr. Robert Fortescue Fox, a physician of the fifth generation of the medical Fox family, said:

> The calling of medicine seems to approach what I conceive to be the chief purpose of Friends, to work for the restoration of harmony in the world. . . . Medical education, which was once almost a priestly office, has become a very long and arduous training in exact branches of medical activity. We see it not only in the hospital and in the daily and nightly routine of the practitioner, but in those who give up their lives in tropical swamps, or in laboratories almost as deadly, in an effort, which has become one long instinctive endeavor, for the prevention and cure of diseases. I sometimes wonder whether the Society of Friends has appreciated at its real value knowledge that has been gained at such a price and which is informed by such a steadfast spirit of service. . . . At its best and highest it is like the gifts of Heaven, for they are shared by the evil and the good, that mortals may have life and have it more abundantly.

Dr. Howard E. Collier, general practitioner and advocate of spiritual healing, in his chapter on health and healing in John Kavanaugh's book *The Quaker Approach* wrote:

> Two simple but profound insights lie at the heart of Quakerism and produce the special characteristics of the typical Quaker approach to health and healing, namely: the affirmation of the unity of all life experience; and the affirmation that the experimental way is the only royal road to a knowledge of truth, right, and conduct. . . . In the final analysis the springs of positive health and the roots of preventive medicine are deeply buried in the life of the spirit and of religion. To me, at least, it is clear that there is no other source from which a sufficiency of steady enduring motive and power can be derived. Therefore, the doctor must say to everyone that positive health requires the coordinated and balanced culture of body, mind, and spirit.

Common Denominators of This Heritage and Their Genesis

What, then, are the common denominators of Quaker belief and action in our profession over these three centuries? The important beliefs may be summarized in two statements: 1) that a caring, loving God (as brought to us in the Christian message) gives unity to all life and that His spirit is potentially present in every human being; 2) that truth must continually be searched for experimentally to the end that this Divine Power may become manifest in all men. The actions that derive from these beliefs are: a) to heal, relieve, or comfort each patient in body, mind, and spirit; b) to experiment, to understand, to increase our skills in the search for truth that will enhance our abilities to promote the healing powers of God; c) to strive to improve the quality of the lives of all men. These beliefs and actions by no means are limited to doctors who are Quakers, but they *are* our heritage of Quaker achievement in the art and science of healing.

How did medical members of the Society of Friends come to be so strongly imbued with these beliefs and so well known for the actions that stemmed from them? In the first century of Quakerism the free-thinking, independent, nonconformism of the early Friends, at a time when most educational and professional opportunities of the Establishment were closed to them, combined with the emphasis on integrity and the innate value of each human life, led many of them to a life of service in medicine and the healing arts. And, being "seekers after truth," they were interested in many aspects of life beyond the confines of medicine. In the succeeding two centuries Quakers have continued to exercise this experimental approach, in combination with their spiritual concern, to the pragmatic end that the life and health of their fellowmen might be improved.

Science and Religion—Quaker Scientists in Other Fields

Quaker physicians and scientists have also contributed theoretically to the great problems and quandaries that lie at the interface of religion and science. The Society of Friends in Great Britain and America has contributed far more than its proportional share of outstanding scientists in nonmedical, as well as in medical, fields. To name a few such nonmedical Quaker scientists in Britain, one can begin with ***John Dalton*** (1766-1844), the chemist and physicist who gave us the periodic atomic table, and go on to ***Sylvanus P. Thompson*** (1851-1916), physicist and teacher of mathematics; ***Sir Arthur Eddington*** (1882-1944), astrophysicist and professor of astronomy at Cambridge; and ***Dame Kathleen Lonsdale*** (1903-1971), crystallographer at the University of London and the first woman scientist to be elected to the Royal Society, to be president of the British Association for the Advancement of Science,and to be made a dame for her scientific achievements. The latter three scientists gave Swarthmore Lectures before the London Yearly Meeting: Thompson, 1915, "The Quest for Truth"; Eddington, 1929, "Science and the Unseen World"; and Lonsdale, 1953, "Removing the Causes of War." All three of these scientists were firm believers in the spiritual life and the experimental approach to truth, but they stressed the limitations of the methods of science in making the approach to the world of values. Some Quaker scientists and doctors have centered their religious life on the divinity of Christ, some on the message of love brought by a wise but not necessarily divine Jesus, some on the mystical evolutionary force of whose process we and our universe are a part, and some, perhaps, have been frankly agnostic. The scope of diversity of belief and action of scientists and doctors in the Society of Friends has been explored by Richard Sutton, American Quaker physicist, in his Ward Lecture, "Quaker Scientists," at Guilford College in 1962 and more recently by David Murray-Rust in his "God in the Universe" at Woodbrooke in 1973.

The Quaker doctors whom we have reviewed have shared this diversity of belief. But most Quaker scientists and physicians appear to have based their lives on the central belief that a caring God gives unity to all life, is potentially present in all men, and must continually be sought for to give strength to one's daily actions. This belief surely lies at the heart of the Quaker heritage in science as well as in medicine.

The Future

"The past is prologue"; how are we to apply this Quaker medical heritage to meeting the challenges of today and tomorrow? As indicated in the introduction, the human predicament has never been more complex and precarious than it is today, faced as we are with the general threats of nuclear destruction, political violence, overpopulation, starvation, environmental pollution, maldistribution of the world's limited resources, and the medical and socio-economic problems of the grossly inadequate distribution of health care. In these circumstances doctors must be both able healers of the sick and responsible citizens of the world; surely our Quaker heritage has a contribution to make to such roles. Does not the search for answers to these great dilemmas "require the recognition that love—in the largest sense of its mystical power—and all the consequences that flow from it, is a necessary ingredient of the whole man and of the abundant life" for all men? We who are Quaker physicians and healers have a great responsibility to carry forward this precious heritage from the past to apply it to the building of the Kingdom of God today and in the future.

SELECTED REFERENCES

SECOND HALF OF THE SEVENTEENTH CENTURY

Cadbury, Henry J., ed. *George Fox's "Book of Miracles."* Cambridge: Cambridge University Press, 1948.

Jones, G. R. "Welshmen and Medicine—An Historical Review." *J. Roy. Coll. Phycns.* 10(1976):303-315.

Lloyd, Humphrey. *The Quaker Lloyds in the Industrial Revolution.* London: Hutchinson, 1975.

Nickalls, John L., ed. *The Journal of George Fox,* pp. 631-632. London: Religious Society of Friends, 1975.

Radbill, S. X. "Medicine in 1776: Colonial and Revolutionary Medicine in Philadelphia." *Trans. and Stud., Coll. Physicians Phila.* 44(2)(1976):1.

THE EIGHTEENTH CENTURY

Abraham, J. Johnston. *Lettsom: His Life, Times, Friends, and Descendants.* London: William Heinemann, 1933.

Booth, C. C. "William Hillary: A Pupil of Boerhaave." *Med. Hist.* 7(1963):297.

———. "Robert Willan, M.D., F.R.S., F.S.A." *Brit. J. Derm.* 80(1968):459.

———. "Doctors from the Yorkshire Dales." *Proc. XXIII Congress Hist. Med.,* (London, 2-9 Sept. 1972), 998-1001.

Corner, Betsy C., and Christopher C. Booth, eds. *Chain of Friendship: Selected Letters of Dr. Fothergill of London, 1735-1780.* Cambridge, Mass.: Harvard Univ. Press, 1971.

Curtis, Wm. Hugh. *A Quaker Doctor and Naturalist in the 19th Century.* London: Bannisdale Press, 1961.

Elkinton, J. R. "Betty Fothergill and Her 'Uncle Doctor': An Intimate Glimpse of Dr. John Fothergill." *Ann. Intern. Med.* 85(1976):637.

Fox, R. Hingston. *Dr. John Fothergill and His Friends: Chapters in Eighteenth Century Life.* London: Macmillan and Co., 1919.

Packard, Francis R. *Some Account of the Pennsylvania Hospital, From its First Rise to the Beginning of the Year 1938.* Philadelphia: Engle Press, 1938.

Raistrick, Arthur. *Quakers in Science and Industry: Being an Account of the Quaker Contributions to Science and Industry During the 17th and 18th Centuries.* Newton Abbot: David and Charles, 1968.

Sessions, W. K., and E. M. Sessions. *The Tukes of York in the 17th, 18th, and 19th Centuries.* York: Wm. Sessions, 1971.

EARLY AND MID-NINETEENTH CENTURY

Godlee, Sir Rickman John. *Lord Lister.* London: Macmillan and Co., 1917.

Talbott, J. H. "Thomas Young (1773-1829), Philologist, Ophthalmologist, Egyptologist." *J. Am. Med. Assoc.* 194(1965):555.

———. "Sir Jonathan Hutchinson (1828-1913). *J. Am. Med. Assoc.* 188(1964): 998.

———. "Sir Francis Galton (1822-1911), Statistician of Eugenics." *J. Am. Med. Assoc.* 194(1965):666.

LATTER NINETEENTH AND EARLY TWENTIETH CENTURIES

Cadbury, William Warder, and Mary Hoxie Jones. *At the Point of a Lancet: One Hundred Years of the Canton Hospital 1835-1935.* Shanghai: Kelly and Walch, 1935.

Crosfield, A. J., and G. Crosfield. *A Man in Shining Armour: Dr. William Wilson of Madagascar.* London: Headley Bros.

Davidson, R. J., and I. Mason. *Life in West China.* London: Headley Bros., 1905.

The Friend, 14 March 1924. Obituary for Ann E. Clark.

The Friend, 24 October 1958. Obituary for W. Henry Davidson.

The Friend, 2 May 1924. Obituary for R. Hingston Fox.

The Friend, 28 June 1940. Obituary for Robert Fortescue Fox.

The Friend, 14 December 1962. Obituary for Lucy E. Harris.

The Friend, 27 March 1925. Obituary for Mary D. Sturge.

Taylor, Robert C. *Dr. E. Claude Taylor.* Gloucester: John Bellows, 1950.

Wood, H. G. *Henry T. Hodgkin: A Memoir.* London: Student Christian Movement Press, 1937.

TWENTIETH CENTURY

Brain, W. Russell. *Man, Society, and Religion.* London: Geo. Allen and Unwin, 1944.

Cadbury, H. J.; L. K. Cleveland; J. D. Cobb; E. C. Corkey; R. L. Day; J. W. Eliot; J. R. Elkinton; J. Stokes, Jr.; J. Abrahamson; H. Abrahamson; H. L. Jennings. *Who Shall Live? Man's Control over Birth and Death. A Report Prepared for the American Friends Service Committee.* New York: Hill and Wang, 1970.

Collier, Howard E. *Experiment with a Life.* London: Friends Home Service Committee, 1953.

———. "Health and Healing." In *The Quaker Approach,* edited by John Kavanaugh. New York: G. P. Putnam's Sons, 1953.

Court, Donald. "A Scientific Age and a Declining Church: What Has a Friend to Say?" *The Friend* (24 September 1965).

Davies, A. Tegla. *Friends Ambulance Unit.* London: Geo. Allen and Unwin, 1947.

Elkinton, J. R. "Friends Medical Society." *Friends Journal* (15 May 1967).

———. "Joseph Stokes, Jr., Physician to Children, Friend of Man." *Medical Affairs* (Univ. of Penna.) (Spring 1972):20-23.

Fox, Theodore F. "The Purposes of Medicine." *Lancet* 2(1965):801.

Franklin, Kenneth J. *Joseph Barcroft 1872-1947.* Oxford: Blackwell, 1953.

The Friend, 13 January 1967. Obituary for W. Russell Brain.

The Friend, 4 March 1977. Obituaries for Cuthbert and Ethel Dukes.

The Friend, 1 or 8 July 1955. Obituary for Henry T. Gillett.

The Friend, 8 July 1955. Obituary for Henry T. Gillett.

The Friend, 6 May 1955. Obituary for Egbert Coleby Morland.

The Friend, 4 June 1948. Obituary for George Newman.

The Friend, 11 August 1972. Obituary for Lionel S. Penrose.

Greenwood, John Ormerod. *Quaker Encounters.* Vol. 1. Friends and Relief. York: William Sessions, 1975.

Heron, Alastair, ed. *Towards a Quaker View of Sex.* London: Friends Home Service Committee, 1963.

Lamerton, R. *The Care of the Dying.* London: Priory Press, 1975.

The Lancet, 19 February 1977. Obituary for Cuthbert Esquire Dukes.

The Lancet, 7 May 1955. Obituary for Egbert Coleby Morland.

Milligan, Edward, ed. *The Past Is Prologue: 100 Years of Quaker Overseas Work, 1868-1968.* London: Friends Service Council, 1968.

Newman, Sir George. *Quaker Profiles.* London: Bannisdale Press, 1946.

Scott, Richenda C. *Quakers in Russia.* London: Michael Joseph, 1964.

Talham, M., and J. E. Miles, eds. *The Friends Ambulance Unit 1914-1919.* London: Swarthmore Press, 1920.

Timbres, Harry, and Rebecca Timbres. *We Didn't Ask Utopia: A Quaker Family in Soviet Russia.* New York: Prentice-Hall, 1939.

CONCLUDING DISCUSSION

Eddington, Arthur S. *Science and the Unseen World.* London, New York: Macmillan Co., 1929.

Lonsdale, Kathleen. *The Christian Life—Lived Experimentally.* Edited by James Hough. London: Friends Home Service Committee, 1976.

Murray-Rust, David. "God in the Universe: A Twentieth-Century Quaker Looks at Science and Theology." *Woodbrooke Occasional Papers* 3. London: Friends Home Service Committee, 1973.

———. "Scientific Man and Sincere Friend: Sylvanus P. Thompson." *Friends Quarterly* 18(1974):299.

Sutton, Richard. "Quaker Scientists." 13th Ward Lecture, Guilford College, North Carolina, 19 October 1962.

Continued from page 12. (Section added in 1986)

A Quaker Hospital in Ireland

DURING the Yearly Meeting of Irish Friends at Dublin, in 1805, so read the minutes, it was resolved "to establish an institution . . . for the accommodation of Friends who may be afflicted with disorders of the mind," and that "there will be peculiar privileges for poor Friends." By 1807 over 777 Pounds had been subscribed. Rather than erect a new building, a suitable one, called *Bloomfield* was bought, at Donnybrook, near Dublin. By 1811 patients were being cared for and rules for management had been adopted. Almost from the beginning, if there were beds not occupied by Friends, non-members were admitted. Irish Friends, typically frugal, wished to keep the income up. Even so, fees were nearly always below expenditure. The difference was made up by contributions.

The management rules were last amended in 1891. At an "Extraordinary General Meeting" in 1963, the rule amended in 1891 was affirmed, that each donation of 100 Pounds from a Meeting, or one of 25 Pounds from an individual Friend, entitled each Meeting or Friend to nominate one poor Quaker patient at a time, "on the lowest terms of admission." So the hospital's charitable purpose was preserved.

According to a letter from the Medical Superintendent, John L. England, in 1980 the hospital (still called *Bloomfield)* was receiving patients as it had for over 170 years. There were in that year 53 patients in residence, with additional accommmodation for 35 elderly people who were still active and not confused.

ACKNOWLEDGMENTS

For information and assistance I am indebted to Esther Williams, Woodbrooke Library; Edward H. Milligan and Malcolm Thomas, Friends House Library; Professor Christopher C. Booth; and Horace G. Alexander. For critical reading of the manuscript as well as for additional information I am grateful to Dr. Robert C. Taylor, Christopher B. and Hannah Taylor, Sir Theodore Fox, Dorothea Rustomjee, Professor Donald Court, and Mary Hoxie Jones; and to my wife, Teresa (Sturge) Elkinton, as always, for her encouragement, critical comment, and, not the least, patience. For any errors of commission or omission, however, I alone am responsible.

To Ackworth School I am indebted for permission to photograph the Wedgwood bust of Dr. John Fothergill and to the *Annals of Internal Medicine* for permission to republish the picture; to the Pennsylvania Hospital I am grateful for the picture of the early Hospital.

J.R.E.

INDEX

XYZ